Copyright 2020 by George Brooks -All rights reserved.

No part of this book may be reproduced or transmitted in any form or by any means, electronic or mechanical, including photocopying and recording, or by any information storage and retrieval system, without permission in writing from the publisher. This is a work of fiction. Names, places, characters and incidents are either the product of the author's imagination or are used fictitiously, and any resemblance to any actual persons, living or dead, organizations, events or locales is entirely coincidental. The unauthorized reproduction or distribution of this copyrighted work is ilegal.

Disclaimer Notice:

Please note the information contained within this document is for educational and entertainment purposes only. All effort has been executed to present accurate, up to date, reliable, complete information. No warranties of any kind are declared or implied. Readers acknowledge that the author is not engaged in the rendering of legal, financial, medical, or professional advice. The content within this book has been derived from various sources. Please consult a licensed professional before attempting any techniques outlined in this book.

By reading this document, the reader agrees that under no circumstances is the author responsible for any losses, direct or indirect, that are incurred as a result of the use of the information contained within this document, including, but not limited to, errors, omissions, or inaccuracies.

CONTENTS

Introduction 5
Breakfast 6
    Banana Walnut Baked Oatmeal 6
    Easy-Peasy Hash Browns 7
    Egg-Stuffed Tomatoes 8
    Grain-Free Pumpkin Pancakes 9
    Peanut Butter Granola 10
    Grain-Free Sweet Potato Waffles 11
    Asparagus Mushroom Frittata 12
    Apple Cinnamon Bars 13
    Banana Almond Butter Muffins 14
    Sweet Potato Oat Bars 15
    Egg-Stuffed Sweet Potatoes 16
    Pumpkin Spice Baked Oatmeal 17
    Vegetable Egg Hash 18
    Oatmeal Pancakes 19
    Spinach and Feta Egg Cups 20
    Savory Chickpea Pancakes 21
    Huevos Rancheros 22
    Cinnamon Apple Stuffed Sweet Potatoes 23
    Sweet Potato Hash 24
    Potato and Bean Hash 25
    Creamy Sweet Potato Bowls 26
Lunch and Dinner 27
    Chicken and Potato Roast 27
    Tex-Mex Chicken and Zucchini 28
    Cuban Chicken and Rice 29
    Cheesy Meatballs 30
    Fish Taco Bowls 31
    Cilantro Lime Salmon 33
    Salmon Patties 34
    Turkey Meatloaf 35
    Chicken with Caramelized Onions and Mushrooms 36
    Chicken Parmesan Pasta Bake 37
    Creamy Potato Soup 38
    White Bean Soup with Lemon 39
    Roasted Tomato Soup 40
    Green Enchilada Soup 41
    Minestrone Soup 42
    Chicken Barley Soup 43
    Carrot Ginger Soup 44
    Seafood Chowder 45
    Creamy Asparagus Soup 46
    Classic Reuben 47

- Vegetable Medley Sandwich ... 48
- Cob Sandwich ... 49
- Chick n' Sandwich ... 50
- Hawaiian Chicken Sandwich ... 51
- Caprese Panini ... 52
- Spicy Tuna Wrap ... 53

Side Dishes ... 54
- Multi-Grain Pilaf with Mushrooms ... 54
- Herb-Scented Rice ... 55
- Toasted Rice with Mushrooms and Thyme ... 56
- Spanish Cauliflower Rice ... 57
- Parmesan Roasted Green Beans ... 58
- Rosemary Sweet Potato Bites ... 59
- Corn and Zucchini with Parmesan ... 60
- Garlic Roasted Broccoli ... 61
- Golden Mashed Potatoes ... 62
- Vibrant Slaw ... 63
- Chinese Chicken Salad ... 64
- Roasted Brussels Sprouts Kale Salad ... 65
- Mediterranean Quinoa Salad ... 66
- Southwestern Salad ... 67
- Autumn Apple Salad ... 68
- Tender Carrot Slaw ... 69

Appetizers and Snacks ... 70
- Cheesy Quinoa Bites ... 70
- Bruschetta ... 71
- Cashew Chicken Lettuce Wraps ... 72
- Smoked Salmon Tea Sandwiches ... 73
- Creamy Cucumber Dill Bites ... 74
- Garlic Chili Edamame ... 75
- Mini Avocado Hummus Quesadillas ... 76
- Deviled Eggs ... 77
- Sweet and Spicy Cauliflower ... 78

Breads ... 79
- Whole-Wheat Sandwich Bread ... 79
- Pumpernickel Bread ... 80
- Gluten-Free Sandwich Bread ... 81
- Quinoa Protein Bread ... 83
- Zucchini Bread ... 84
- Whole-Grain Cornbread ... 85

Sauces, Gravies, and Marinades ... 86
- Date Paste ... 86
- Cashew Queso Sauce ... 87
- Chimichurri Sauce ... 88
- Mango Habanero Sauce ... 89

- Stir-Fry Sauce 90
- Creamy Cauliflower Alfredo Sauce 91
- Sweet and Spicy Marinade 92
- Fresh Greek Marinade 93
- Brown Rice Gravy 94
- Dairy-Free Tzatziki Sauce 95
- Japanese Ginger Salad Dressing 96
- Strawberry Poppy Seed Vinaigrette 97
- Green Goddess Salad Dressing 98
- Thousand Island Dressing 99
- Simple Mayonnaise 100

Beverages 101
- Green Ginger Smoothie 101
- Chocolate Banana Smoothie 102
- Tropical Detox Smoothie 103
- Peach Cobbler Smoothie 104
- Matcha Antioxidant Smoothie 105
- Chocolate Pudding Shake 106
- Coffee Breakfast Smoothie 107
- Apple Pie Protein Smoothie 108
- Lemonade Sunshine Shake 109
- Summer Watermelon Cooler 110
- ACV Detox Tea 111

Desserts 112
- Gluten-Free Lemon Bars 112
- Cherry Crisp 113
- Peanut Butter Banana Oatmeal Cookies 114
- Zucchini Brownies 115

Introduction

The anti-inflammatory diet is a powerful way to take your health and weight into your own hands. Rather than dieting and trying to lose weight, only to experience extreme weight fluctuations back and forth, sleep disorders, chronic pain, high blood pressure, sleep disorders, and countless other problems, you can find a new way. By choosing anti-inflammatory ingredients, rather than the pro-inflammatory foods many of us eat on a day-to-day basis, you can rewrite your body's health and healing ability. You can lower the chronic inflammation that worsens and cause all of these problems and more. The truth is that many of the worst illnesses that are plaguing the modern world are based in inflammation. But you can do something about that. You are not helpless.

In *The Anti-Inflammatory Diet Cookbook*, you will be provided with over one-hundred recipes to help you successfully lower your chronic inflammation and start a new healthier, and happier way of life. You can finally find the answer to the success that you have been looking for. But you are not alone on this journey. In my other book, *The Anti-Inflammatory Diet Action Plan*, you can gain the information you need to start and follow the anti-inflammatory diet easily, including a thirty-day menu plan and bonus recipes!

When reading, please keep in mind that I am not a doctor, and this book is not making medical claims or practicing medicine. You should always discuss anything related to medicine, health, or diet with your doctor before making any changes. This applies to all of the information in this book.

Breakfast

Banana Walnut Baked Oatmeal

This baked oatmeal is so delicious, you will feel like you are spoiling yourself with dessert! If you have allergies to gluten, then be sure to use certified gluten-free oats. You can also replace the walnuts with other nut varieties or remove them entirely if you have nut allergies.

The Servings: 9
The Time to Prepare/Cook: 40 minutes
The Calories: 291
The Ingredients:
Rolled oats – 2.25 cups
Banana, mashed – 1 cup
Eggs – 2
Date paste – 2 tablespoons
Soybean oil – 3 tablespoons
Almond milk, unsweetened – 1 cup
Vanilla extract – 1 teaspoon
Sea salt – 0.5 teaspoon
Cinnamon – 1 teaspoon
Baking powder – 1 teaspoon
Walnuts, chopped – 0.5 cup

The Instructions:
1. Warm your oven to a temperature of Fahrenheit 350 degrees and either grease or line an eight-by-eight baking dish with kitchen parchment to prevent sticking.
2. In a kitchen bowl, whisk together the date paste with the mashed banana, almond milk, eggs, soybean oil, and vanilla. Whisk this mixture until the date paste is completely combined into the other ingredients without clumps. But, clumps from the mashed banana are okay.
3. Stir the Rolled oats, cinnamon, sea salt, and baking powder into the banana mixture, and then gently fold in your chopped walnuts.
4. Once your banana walnut oats are combined, spread the mixture into the bottom of your prepared baking pan and set the dish in the center of your hot oven. Allow it to bake until the oats are golden in color and set, about thirty to thirty-five minutes. Remove the dish of baked oatmeal from the oven and allow it to cool for at least five minutes before serving. Enjoy alone, or with fresh fruit and yogurt.

Easy-Peasy Hash Browns

Have you ever struggled to make hash browns because they always seem to either stick, burn, or even come out partially raw? Thankfully, hash browns no longer have to be such a chore to make! With this recipe, they are cooked in a waffle iron, making them easy-peasy.

The Servings: 3
The Time to Prepare/Cook: 35 minutes
The Calories: 209
The Ingredients:
Shredded hash browns, frozen – 1 pound
Eggs – 2
Sea salt – 0.5 teaspoon
Garlic powder – 0.5 teaspoon
Onion powder – 0.5 teaspoon
Black pepper, ground – 0.125 teaspoon
Extra virgin olive oil – 1 tablespoon
The Instructions:
1. Start by warming up your waffle iron.
2. In a kitchen bowl whisk together the eggs to break them down, and then add in the remaining ingredients. Fold them all together until the potato is evenly coated by the egg and seasonings.
3. Grease your waffle iron and spread one-third of the hash brown mixture onto it. Close it and allow the potatoes to cook inside until golden-brown, about twelve to fifteen minutes. Once down, gently remove the hash brown using a fork and then continue to cook another third of the mixture and then the final third.
4. You can store the cooked hash browns in the fridge and then reheat them in the waffle iron or in the oven to get them crispy again later on.

Egg-Stuffed Tomatoes

These eggs are nestled into tomatoes and roasted, giving them amazing flavor and texture. This dish is delicious, healthy, and perfect for fans of Italian cuisine.

The Servings: 2
The Time to Prepare/Cook: 40 minutes
The Calories: 220
The Ingredients:
Tomatoes, large, ripe – 2
Eggs – 2
Parmesan cheese, shredded – 0.25 cup
Green onion, sliced – 3
Garlic, minced – 2 cloves
Parsley, fresh – 1 tablespoon
Sea salt – 0.5 teaspoon
Extra virgin olive oil – 1 tablespoon
Black pepper, ground – 0.5 teaspoon

The Instructions:
1. Warm your oven to Fahrenheit 350 degrees and prepare an oven-safe skillet for cooking.
2. On a cutting board, slice a round off the top of the tomato surrounding the stem. Use a spoon to gently scoop inside the tomato where you cut it and remove the seeds of the fruit, discarding them. You should be left with a casing of the tomato fruit, minus the excess liquid and seeds.
3. In a kitchen mixing dish, combine your sea salt, black pepper, and the fresh parsley. Once combined, sprinkle half of the mixture into each tomato, using your hand or a spoon to spread the seasonings around the inside wall of the tomato.
4. In the skillet, heat the garlic and green onions in the olive oil over medium until soft and fragrant—about four to five minutes. Once done, stir in the Parmesan cheese and divide the mixture between the two tomatoes, placing it inside. Now that the skillet is empty, transfer the tomatoes from the cutting board into the skillet. Lastly, crack one egg into each tomato.
5. Place your skillet with the stuffed tomatoes in the warm oven and allow it to roast until the egg is cooked through, about twenty-five to thirty minutes. Remove the dish of egg-stuffed tomatoes from the oven and serve while warm, either alone or with toasted whole-wheat bread.

Grain-Free Pumpkin Pancakes

These pancakes are great for people who feel best when they consume little or no grains. Remember, the anti-inflammatory diet is all about doing what is best for your body. That means if you feel best eating grains, then continue to eat them. But, if you find that grains increase your inflammation and make you feel ill, then it is best to refrain. The good news is that everyone, whether they eat grains or not, can enjoy these pancakes.

The Servings: 3
The Time to Prepare/Cook: 30 minutes
The Calories: 278
The Ingredients:
Almond flour – 1 cup
Nutmeg, ground – 0.25 teaspoon
Cinnamon, ground – 0.5 teaspoon
Sea salt – 0.5 teaspoon
Baking powder – 1 teaspoon
Baking soda – 1 teaspoon
Soybean oil – 1 tablespoon
Vanilla extract – 1 teaspoon
Apple cider vinegar – 1 teaspoon
Almond milk, unsweetened – 0.75 cup
Eggs – 1
Pumpkin puree – 0.75 cup
Date paste – 1 tablespoon

The Instructions:
1. In a kitchen bowl, whisk together your almond flour, leavening agents, and spices. Add in the remaining ingredients, whisking just until completely combined, being careful to not over mix the batter, as that will deflate the leavening.
2. Warm an electric griddle or non-stick skillet over medium. Once hot, grease the griddle and then ladle the pancake batter onto the heat. Pancakes cook best if each pancake consists of two to three tablespoons of batter. Be sure to not place them too closely together, or it will be difficult to flip them.
3. All the pancakes to cook until they bubble and the first side is golden-brown, and then flip them carefully—about three minutes. Flip the grain-free pumpkin pancakes and cook the other side for a few minutes and then remove the pancakes from the griddle. Continue cooking any batter you have remaining.
4. Serve the pancakes hot with your favorite toppings, such as yogurt and fresh berries, fruit compote, or Lakanto's monk fruit maple-flavored syrup.

Peanut Butter Granola

This granola is super tasty and will feel just like eating dessert! If you have allergies, you can replace the peanut butter with almond butter, use gluten-free oats, or leave out the chocolate. When using chocolate chips, I recommend Lily's brand, as it is naturally sugar-free by using stevia as a sweetener.

The Servings: 8
The Time to Prepare/Cook: 25 minutes
The Calories: 250
The Ingredients:
Rolled oats – 2 cups
Cinnamon – 0.5 teaspoon
Peanut butter, natural with salt – 0.5 cup
Date paste – 1.5 tablespoons
Lily's dark chocolate chips – 0.5 cup
The Instructions:
1. Warm the oven to Fahrenheit 300 degrees and line a baking sheet with kitchen parchment or a silicone kitchen mat.
2. In a bowl, whisk together the date paste, cinnamon, and peanut butter to combine, and then add in the oats, tossing until the oats are fully coated. Spread this sweetened and spiced mixture evenly over the baking sheet in a thin layer.
3. Place the peanut butter granola in the oven and bake for twenty minutes, giving it a good stir halfway through the cooking time to prevent uneven cooking and burning.
4. Remove the granola from the oven and allow it to cool to room temperature before tossing in the chocolate chips. Transfer the peanut butter granola to an airtight container to store until use.

Grain-Free Sweet Potato Waffles

These sweet potato waffles are delicious and extremely healthy, as they aren't filled up with a bunch of flours—but instead are primarily sweet potatoes. This means you get all the health benefits of the sweet potato while also being able to enjoy a delicious waffle.

The Servings: 2
The Time to Prepare/Cook: 15 minutes
The Calories: 364
The Ingredients:
Sweet potatoes, shredded – 3 cups
Coconut flour – 2 tablespoons
Arrowroot – 1 tablespoon
Eggs – 2
Soybean oil – 1 tablespoon
Cinnamon, ground – 0.5 teaspoon
Nutmeg, ground – 0.25 teaspoon
Sea salt – 0.25 teaspoon
Date paste – 1 tablespoon

The Instructions:
1. Before mixing up your waffles, start by warming up your waffle iron.
2. In a bowl, whisk together the eggs, soybean oil, and date paste until combined. Add in the remaining ingredients and stir until all of the ingredients are evenly distributed.
3. Grease your heated waffle iron and add in some of your batter. Closer the iron and let your waffle to cook until golden-brown, about six to seven minutes. Once done, remove the waffle with a fork and then cook the second half of the batter in the same way.
4. Serve the grain-free sweet potato waffles hot with your favorite toppings, such as yogurt and fresh berries, fruit compote, or Lakanto's monk fruit maple-flavored syrup.

Asparagus Mushroom Frittata

This is the perfect single-serving frittata to start out your day with! Whether it is a workday or the weekend, this frittata will keep you fueled and energized with all the nutrients you need to start the day off right.

The Servings: 1
The Time to Prepare/Cook:
The Calories: 333
The Ingredients:
Eggs – 2
Asparagus spears – 5
Water – 1 tablespoon
Extra virgin olive oil – 1 tablespoon
Button mushrooms, sliced – 3
Sea salt – pinch
Green onion, chopped – 1
Goat cheese, semi-soft – 2 tablespoons
The Instructions:
1. Warm your oven on the broiler setting while you prepare your frittata. Prepare your vegetables, discarding the tough end on the asparagus spears and then slicing the spears into bite-sized pieces.
2. Grease a seven to eight-inch oven-safe skillet and place it over medium heat. Add in the mushrooms and allow them to sauté for two minutes before adding in the asparagus and cooking for an additional two minutes. Once they are done sautéing, evenly distribute the vegetables over the bottom of the pan.
3. In a small kitchen mixing dish, whisk together the eggs, water, and sea salt and then pour it over the sautéed vegetables. Sprinkle the chopped green onion and crumbled goat cheese over the top of the frittata.
4. Allow the pan to continue cooking on the stove in this way without being disturbed until the scrambled eggs from the frittata begin to set around the edges and pull away from the sides of the pan. Carefully, lift the pan and turn it in gentle circular motions so that the egg cooks evenly.
5. Transfer your frittata to the oven, cooking under the boiler until the egg is fully cooked, another two to three minutes. Keep a close eye on the egg for your frittata, so that it doesn't over cook. Remove it from the oven as soon as it is done, transfer the frittata to a plate, and enjoy while hot.

Apple Cinnamon Bars

These apple cinnamon bars are a great option to make ahead and store for an on-the-go breakfast. Whether you simply want to enjoy your mornings relaxing without cooking or if you have to eat on the road, you will find these bars to be a great option! Remember, if you are sensitive to gluten, then use gluten-free oats.

The Servings: 4
The Time to Prepare/Cook: 35 minutes
The Calories: 250
The Ingredients:
Oats – 1 cup
Cinnamon, ground – 1 teaspoon
Baking powder – 0.5 teaspoon
Baking soda – 0.5 teaspoon
Vanilla extract – 1 teaspoon
Sea salt – 0.125 teaspoon
Lakanto monk fruit sweetener – 3 tablespoons
Apple, peeled and diced – 1
Yogurt, plain – 3 tablespoons
Soybean oil – 1 tablespoon
Eggs – 2

The Instructions:
1. Warm your oven to Fahrenheit 350 degrees and line an eight-by-eight inch square baking dish with kitchen parchment.
2. In a blender, add three-quarters of your oats and the remaining ingredients. Blend until combined and then use a spatula to stir in the last remaining oats. Pour the mixture into your prepared baking dish and then place it in the center of the oven to bake until the apple cinnamon bars are cooked through, about twenty-five to thirty minutes. The bars are ready when a knife or toothpick is inserted and removed cleanly.
3. Remove the apple cinnamon bar pan from the oven and allow the bars to cool completely before slicing them and chilling in the fridge. While you can eat these bars at room temperature, they are best when you allow them to chill for a while first.

Banana Almond Butter Muffins

Muffins are a great breakfast option, as they can easily be made in advance, cause little mess, and are portable. But most muffins are full of refined flours, sugars, and oils, making them terrible for your health. Thankfully, these are made with delicious and healthy ingredients, such as oats, almond butter, and bananas. If you don't have any oat flour, you can make some simply by blending gluten-free oats in your food processing device or stand blender until it forms a fine meal.

The Servings: 6
The Time to Prepare/Cook: 30 minutes
The Calories: 322
The Ingredients:
Oat flour – 1 cup
Sea salt – 0.25 teaspoon
Cinnamon, ground – 0.5 teaspoon
Baking powder – 1 teaspoon
Almond butter – 0.75 cup
Banana, mashed – 1 cup
Almond milk, unsweetened – 0.5 tablespoon
Vanilla extract – 2 teaspoons
Eggs – 2
Lakanto monk fruit sweetener – 0.25 cup

The Instructions:
1. Warm your oven to Fahrenheit 350 degrees and line a muffin tin with paper liners or grease it if you would rather.
2. In a kitchen bowl, whisk together your mashed banana with the almond butter, unsweetened almond milk, eggs, vanilla extract, and monk fruit sweetener. In a separate kitchen mixing dish, combine together the oat flour, spices, and baking powder. Once the flour mixture is fully combined, pour it into the bowl with the mashed banana and fold both the almond butter/banana mixture and the oat flour mixtures together just until combined.
3. Divide the muffin batter between the twelve paper liners, filling each muffin cavity about three-quarters of the way full. Place the banana almond butter muffins tin in the middle of your hot oven and allow them to cook until set and cooked through. They are done once a toothpick is pricked inside the center and removed cleanly. This should take about twenty to twenty-five minutes.
4. Allow the banana almond butter muffins to cool before serving, and then enjoy.

Sweet Potato Oat Bars

These bars are a tasty way to start out the morning and they are also versatile! While I like to add in dried coconut and pecans, you can add in whatever nuts or unsweetened dried fruit you like. When using protein powder, be sure that you use a pure healthy variety without added ingredients. For instance, you can get some that are nothing but egg whites or soybean isolate.

The Servings: 6
The Time to Prepare/Cook: 35 minutes
The Calories: 226
The Ingredients:
Sweet potato, cooked, mashed – 1 cup
Almond milk, unsweetened – 0.75 cup
Egg – 1
Date paste – 1.5 tablespoons
Vanilla extract – 1.5 teaspoons
Baking soda – 1 teaspoon
Cinnamon, ground – 1 teaspoon
Cloves, ground – 0.25 teaspoon
Nutmeg, ground – 0.5 teaspoon
Ginger, ground – 0.5 teaspoon
Flaxseed, ground – 2 tablespoons
Protein powder – 1 serving
Coconut flour – 0.25 cup
Oat flour – 1 cup
Dried coconut, unsweetened – 0.25 cup
Pecans, chopped – 0.25 cup

The Instructions:
1. Warm the oven to Fahrenheit 375 degrees and line a square eight-by-eight inch baking dish with kitchen parchment. You want to leave some parchment paper hanging over the sides of the pan for lifting once the bars are done baking.
2. Into your stand blender, add all of the ingredients for the sweet potato oat bars except for the dried coconut and chopped pecans. Allow the mixture to pulse for a few moments until the mixture is smooth and then stop the blender. You may need to scrape the sides of the blender down and then blend again.
3. Pour the coconut and pecans into the batter and then stir them in with a spatula. Do not blend the mixture again, as you don't want these pieces blended. Pour the sweet potato oat bar mixture into your prepared pan and spread it out.
4. Place your sweet potato oat bar dish in the middle of your oven and allow it to bake until the bars are set through, about twenty-two to twenty-five minutes. Remove the pan from the oven. Set a wire cooling rack next to the baking dish and then gently life the kitchen parchment by the overhang and carefully lift it from the dish and onto the wire rack to cool. Allow the sweet potato oat bars to cool completely before slicing.

Egg-Stuffed Sweet Potatoes

This is a delicious sweet and savory breakfast. You will love how the sweet potato and egg combine to create an irresistible flavor. These are best made and served fresh from the oven, while the egg is still tender. But you can make them quickly if you keep cooked sweet potatoes ready in the fridge so that you can make this dish at a moment's notice.

The Servings: 1
The Time to Prepare/Cook: 25 minutes
The Calories: 386
The Ingredients:

Sweet potato, cooked – 1
Eggs, large – 2
Cheddar cheese, shredded – 2 tablespoons
Green onion, sliced – 1
Extra virgin olive oil – 0.5 tablespoon
Button mushroom, diced – 2
Sea salt – 0.25 teaspoon

The Instructions:

1. Warm your oven to Fahrenheit 350 degrees and prepare a small baking sheet or dish for the potatoes.
2. Slice the cooked sweet potato in half and place them on the baking sheet. Using a spoon, carefully scoop the potato's orange flesh out of the peel, careful to leave the peel intact without breaking it. Transfer the potato's flesh to a small bowl. Use a fork to mash the meat of the sweet potato in the bowl.
3. Into the sweet potato in the bowl, add the cheddar cheese, green onion, olive oil, and mushrooms. Combine the mixture and then scoop it back into the sweet potato's peel on the baking sheet.
4. Use your spoon to create a crater or well in the center of each potato half, and then crack one egg into each crater. Sprinkle your sea salt over the sweet potato and egg.
5. Place the baking sheet with the potatoes in the oven and allow them to bake until the egg is set to your preference and the potato is hot, about fifteen to twenty minutes. Remove the sheet from the oven and enjoy them fresh and hot.

Pumpkin Spice Baked Oatmeal

Mornings are best when you have a warm cozy meal and can relax. With this oatmeal, even if you don't have much time, you can spend a few minutes relaxing before starting your day. You can even make this oatmeal ahead of time and store it in the fridge, reheating it when you are ready to serve the baked oatmeal. Enjoy it on its own or with a dollop of yogurt.

The Servings: 6
The Time to Prepare/Cook: 35 minutes
The Calories: 262
The Ingredients:
Rolled oats – 1.5 cups
Almond milk, unsweetened – 0.75 cup
Egg – 1
Lakanto monk fruit sweetener – 0.5 cup
Pumpkin puree – 1 cup
Vanilla extract – 1 teaspoon
Pecans, chopped – 0.75 cup
Baking powder – 1 teaspoon
Sea salt – 0.5 teaspoon
Pumpkin pie spice – 1.5 teaspoons

The Instructions:
1. Warm your oven to Fahrenheit 350 degrees and grease an eight-by-eight baking dish.
2. In a bowl, whisk together the rolled oats, almond milk, eggs, and remaining ingredients until the oatmeal batter is fully combined. Pour the pumpkin spiced oatmeal mixture into your greased pan and place it in the center of your oven.
3. Bake your oatmeal until it is golden in color and set, about twenty-five to thirty minutes. Remove the pumpkin spice baked oatmeal from the oven and allow it to cool for five minutes before serving. Enjoy warm alone or with your favorite fruit and yogurt.

Vegetable Egg Hash

This hash is a perfect single pan breakfast that will give you a complete meal. You will love this hash when paired with the fresh eggs cooked to your preference. If you want to make this hash even easier to prepare, you can chop and freeze the vegetables in a large container ahead of time. Then, when you go to prepare your hash you just have to take them out of the freezer, no chopping necessary.

The Servings: 4
The Time to Prepare/Cook: 35 minutes
The Calories: 213
The Ingredients:
Baby new potatoes, quartered – 10 ounces
Zucchini, chopped – 1
Garlic, minced – 2 cloves
Red bell pepper, chopped – 1
Yellow bell pepper, chopped – 1
Green onion, chopped – 2
Extra virgin olive oil – 2 tablespoon
Sea salt – 0.75 teaspoon
Red pepper flakes – 0.5 teaspoon
Eggs, large – 4
Black pepper, ground – 0.25 teaspoon

The Instructions:
1. Allow your quartered potatoes to boil in a large pot of salted water until fork-tender, about six to eight minutes. Drain them off, discarding the water.
2. Add the quartered baby new potatoes to a large skillet along with the bell peppers, zucchini, garlic, and olive oil. Sprinkle the seasonings for the egg hash over the top and then allow the hash to sauté until the vegetables are browned, about eight to ten minutes. Be sure to give the hash a good stir every couple of minutes for even cooking.
3. Once the vegetables are ready, use a spoon to create four craters or wells for the eggs to fit into. Crack the eggs into the craters, with one egg per crater. Place a lid on the skillet and allow the eggs to cook until cooked to your preference, about four to five minutes.
4. Remove the skillet of the vegetable egg hash from the heat, sprinkle the green onions over the top, and enjoy the hash and eggs while hot.

Oatmeal Pancakes

Oatmeal pancakes are a great alternative to regular pancakes, as they have a great nutty flavor and will stick with you longer. Plus, you don't have to worry about refined grains affecting your inflammation! Just remember to use gluten-free oats if you are allergic to gluten.

The Servings: 1
The Time to Prepare/Cook: 10 minutes
The Calories: 395
The Ingredients:
Egg – 1
Rolled oats, ground – 0.5 cup
Almond milk – 2 tablespoons
Baking soda – 0.125 teaspoon
Baking powder – 0.125 teaspoon
Vanilla extract – 1 teaspoon
Date paste – 1 teaspoon
The Instructions:
1. Warm up your non-stick griddle or skillet over medium while you prepare the pancakes.
2. Place the rolled oats into your blender or food processor and pulse until they grind into a fine flour. Add them to a bowl, whisking them with the baking powder and baking soda.
3. In another kitchen bowl, whisk together the egg with almond milk, date paste, and vanilla extract until combined. Add the sweetened egg/almond milk mixture to the oat flour mixture and fold together just until combined.
4. Grease your skillet and then ladle on your pancake batter leaving a bit of room between each pancake. Allow your pancakes to cook for about two to three minutes, until golden-brown and bubbly. Carefully, flip over the pancakes and cook the other side for a couple of minutes until it is golden, as well.
5. Remove your pancakes from the stove and serve them with your choice of fruit, yogurt, compote, or Lakanto's monk fruit maple-flavored syrup.

Spinach and Feta Egg Cups

These delicious egg cups are not only a delicious way to enjoy eggs, they are easy to make, too! While eggs can easily stick and burn to the pan, these are much simpler. Lastly, you can make them several days in advance, storing them in the fridge and then reheating when ready to enjoy—though they're even good cold!

The Servings: 3
The Time to Prepare/Cook: 25 minutes
The Calories: 192
The Ingredients:

Eggs, large – 6
Black pepper, ground – 0.125 teaspoon
Onion powder – 0.25 teaspoon
Garlic powder – 0.25 teaspoon
Feta cheese – 0.33 cup
Baby spinach – 1.5 cups
Sea salt – 0.25 teaspoon

The Instructions:

1. Warm your oven to Fahrenheit 350 degrees, set the rack to the center of the oven, and grease a muffin tin.
2. Divide your baby spinach and feta cheese into the bottom of the twelve muffin cups.
3. In a bowl, whisk together the eggs, sea salt, garlic powder, onion powder, and black pepper until the egg white is fully broken down into the yolk. Pour the egg over the spinach and cheese in the muffin cups, filling the cups three-quarters of the way. Place the baking tin in the oven until the eggs are fully cooked, about eighteen to twenty minutes.
4. Remove the spinach and feta egg cups from the oven and serve warm or allow the eggs to cool completely at room temperature before chilling.

Savory Chickpea Pancakes

These savory pancakes are a great option when you don't want something sweet, but also don't feel like eggs. Enjoy these pancakes best with garnishes of hummus, guacamole, or salsa.

The Servings: 1
The Time to Prepare/Cook: 15 minutes
The Calories: 202
The Ingredients:
Water – 0.5 cup, plus 2 tablespoons
Onion, finely diced – 0.25 cup
Bell pepper, finely diced – 0.25 cup
Chickpea flour – 0.5 cup
Baking powder – 0.25 teaspoon
Sea salt – 0.25 teaspoon
Garlic powder – 0.25 teaspoon
Red pepper flakes – 0.125 teaspoon
Black pepper, ground – 0.125 teaspoon

The Instructions:
1. Warm a ten-inch non-stick skillet over medium while you prepare your chickpea pancake batter.
2. In a kitchen mixing dish, whisk together the chickpea flour with the baking powder and seasonings. Once combined, whisk in the water and whisk it vigorously for fifteen to thirty seconds, to whip a lot of air bubbles into the chickpea batter and breakdown and lumps. Stir in the diced onion and bell pepper.
3. Once the skillet is hot, pour all of the batter into it all at once to create a single large pancake. Move the pan in circular motions to evenly distribute the batter over the entire bottom of the pan, and then let it rest undisturbed.
4. Cook the chickpea pancake until it is set and can easily be flipped without breaking, about five to seven minutes. The bottom of it should be golden-brown. Carefully, flip the savory chickpea pancake with a large spatula and allow the other side to cook for an additional five minutes.
5. Remove the skillet with the savory chickpea pancake from the heat and transfer the pancake to a plate, keeping it whole or slicing it into wedges. Serve with your pick of savory sauces and dips.

Huevos Rancheros

This dish is a popular breakfast originating from rural Mexico. It's great, because it is a complete meal, delicious, easy, and quick to make. In fact, you could serve this any time of the day and enjoy it equally.

The Servings: 3
The Time to Prepare/Cook: 20 minutes
The Calories: 464
The Ingredients:
Eggs – 6
Corn tortillas, small – 6
Refried beans – 1.5 cups
Diced green chilies, canned – 4 ounces
Fore-roasted canned tomatoes – 14.5 ounces
Avocado, sliced – 1
Garlic, minced – 2 cloves
Cilantro, chopped – 0.5 cup
Onion, diced – 0.5
Sea salt – 0.5 teaspoon
Cumin, ground – 0.5 teaspoon
Extra virgin olive oil – 1 teaspoon
Black pepper, ground – 0.25 teaspoon

The Instructions:
1. In a saucepan, allow the fire-roasted tomatoes, green chilies, sea salt, cumin, and black pepper to simmer for five minutes.
2. Meanwhile, sauté the onion and olive oil in a large skillet, adding in the garlic the last minute of cooking—about five minutes in total.
3. Pan-fry your eggs to your desired cooking preference; heat your refried beans, and warm your tortillas.
4. To serve, spoon your refried beans, tomatoes, onions, and eggs over the tortillas. Top with the avocado and cilantro and then enjoy fresh and hot. You can add a little salsa, cheese, or sour cream, if you would like.

Cinnamon Apple Stuffed Sweet Potatoes

This breakfast is so good, that you will feel like you are eating dessert. While it may not have any sweetener, you will be surprised how naturally sweet it is from the apples and sweet potatoes, which become creamy when combined with the almond butter.

The Servings: 4
The Time to Prepare/Cook: 10 minutes
The Calories: 327
The Ingredients:
Sweet potatoes, baked – 4
Red apples, diced – 3
Water – 0.25 cup
Sea salt – pinch
Cinnamon, ground – 1 teaspoon
Cloves, ground – 0.125 teaspoon
Ginger, ground – 0.5 teaspoon
Pecans, chopped – 0.25 cup
Almond butter – 0.25 cup

The Instructions:
1. In a large non-stick skillet combine the apples with the water, sea salt, spices, and pecans. Cover the apples with a tight-fitting lid and allow them to simmer for about five to seven minutes, until tender. The exact time cooking the spiced apples will take will depend on the size of your apple slices and the variety of apple you use.
2. Slice the baked sweet potatoes in half, placing each half on a serving plate. When the apples are done cooking, top the sweet potatoes with them, and then drizzle the almond butter over the top. Serve while still warm.

Sweet Potato Hash

This hash is sweet, savory, and delicious! If you are tight on time in the mornings, you can easily make it ahead of time. Then, when you wake up all you have to do is reheat it in a skillet and throw in an egg, if you want. You can also wash and chop the vegetables ahead of time and then freeze them until ready to cook.

The Servings: 3
The Time to Prepare/Cook: 25 minutes
The Calories: 254
The Ingredients:
Sweet potatoes, diced – 1 pound
Water – 1 cup
Onion, diced – 0.5
Yellow bell pepper, diced – 1
Red bell pepper, diced – 1
Garlic, minced – 2 cloves
Extra virgin olive oil – 2 tablespoons
Sea salt – 0.5 teaspoon
Parsley, chopped – 2 tablespoons
Black pepper, ground – 0.25 teaspoon

The Instructions:
1. Place the sweet potatoes and a cup of water into a large saucepan and cover with a lid, placing the stove to medium-high. Allow the potatoes to cook in this way for ten minutes, stirring them every couple of minutes so that they cook evenly. When ready, discard the water.
2. Transfer the sweet potatoes into a large skillet with the olive oil, giving them a good toss. Pan-fry the potatoes until they start to brown on the edges, about five to six minutes over medium-high.
3. Stir the onion, garlic, and bell pepper into your skillet, until tender with still a little bit of bite, about five minutes. Toss in your sea salt, black pepper, and parsley and remove the dish from the heat to serve. Enjoy alone or with eggs.

Potato and Bean Hash

This hash is great for people who want to reduce their consumption of meat or eggs while still getting all the protein their body requires. The pinto beans perfectly pair with the vegetables and seasonings, so you won't even miss the animal products!

The Servings: 4
The Time to Prepare/Cook: 50 minutes
The Calories: 255
The Ingredients:
Potatoes, diced – 4 cups
Mushrooms, sliced – 0.5 cup
Bell pepper, diced – 1
Zucchini, diced – 1 cup
Yellow squash, diced – 1 cup
Pinto beans, cooked – 1.75 cup
Black pepper, ground – 0.25 teaspoon
Paprika, ground – 0.5 teaspoon
Sea salt – 0.5 teaspoon
Onion powder – 1.5 teaspoons
Garlic powder – 1.5 teaspoon

The Instructions:
1. Warm your oven to Fahrenheit 425 degrees ad line a large aluminum baking sheet with kitchen parchment.
2. Add your diced potatoes onto your baking sheet and toss them with the sea salt and black pepper. Place the seasoned diced potatoes in the oven to roast for twenty-five minutes. Remove the potatoes and give them a good stir.
3. Meanwhile, Stir the remaining ingredients for the hash into a large oven-safe skillet. After you toss the partially roasted potatoes, place the potato pan and the vegetable skillet both in the oven. Allow both portions of the hash to roast for fifteen additional minutes.
4. Remove the pan and skillet from the oven and toss the skillet's contents with the roasted potatoes. Serve alone or with eggs.

Creamy Sweet Potato Bowls

I like to keep sweet potatoes in my fridge at all times so that whenever I get hungry, I can whip up one of these sweet potato bowls. They are irresistible! Feel free to adjust the recipe for your preferences, you may want to use different berries, add in some crunchy seeds and nuts, or coconut flakes.

The Servings: 2
The Time to Prepare/Cook: 7 minutes
The Calories: 306
The Ingredients:
Sweet potato, baked – 2
Almond milk, unsweetened – 0.5 cup
Cinnamon, ground – 0.25 teaspoon
Vanilla extract – 0.5 teaspoon
Flaxseed, ground – 1 tablespoon
Date paste – 1 tablespoon
Almond butter – 2 tablespoons
Blueberries – 0.5 cup

The Instructions:
1. You want your roasted sweet potatoes hot, so if they were previously roasted and chilled, reheat the cooked sweet potatoes in the microwave or oven prior to making your bowls.
2. Remove the sweet potato peel and place the flesh of the potato in a blender along with all of the other sweet potato bowl ingredients except for the blueberries. Pulse it until smooth and creamy, about thirty seconds, and then transfer the contents into a large bowl. Top the bowl with the blueberries, and if you would like, a little extra almond milk. You can even add some granola, nuts, or seeds, if you would like a crunch.

Lunch and Dinner

Chicken and Potato Roast

This classic chicken and potato roast contains only a few staple ingredients that you can easily keep on hand, making it easy to enjoy a delicious home-cooked meal no matter the circumstances. Whether you are looking for a simple comfort dish or hope to impress for date night, you will find that this roast is the perfect go-to meal.

The Servings: 6
The Time to Prepare/Cook: 1 hour
The Calories: 675
The Chicken Ingredients:
Chicken breast, bone-in, skin-on – 6, medium
Garlic, minced – 4 cloves
Sea salt – 2 teaspoons
Rosemary, fresh, chopped – 1 tablespoon
Thyme, fresh, chopped – 1 tablespoon
Lemon zest – 0.5 teaspoon
Black pepper, ground – 0.5 teaspoon
Extra virgin olive oil – 2 tablespoons
Lemon juice – 1 tablespoon
The Potato Ingredients:
Yellow potatoes, small, quartered – 1.5 pounds
Sea salt – 1 teaspoon
Lemon, thinly sliced rounds – 1
Extra virgin olive oil – 2 tablespoons
Black pepper, ground – 0.5 teaspoon
The Instructions:
1. Warm your oven to Fahrenheit 450 degrees. Onto a large baking sheet, place your potatoes and the olive oil and seasoning from their ingredient list. Toss the quartered yellow potatoes in this mixture until they are evenly coated and then spread them out on the baking dish in a single layer. Partially bake the potatoes, placing them in the oven for fifteen minutes.
2. Meanwhile, use a paper towel to pat your chicken breasts dry. Add them into a bowl toss together the chicken breasts with their herbs and seasonings, olive oil, lemon zest, and lemon juice.
3. After you take the roasted yellow potatoes out of the oven, add the chicken breasts to the pan. Press them between the sliced potatoes skin-side facing upward. Place your lemon slices around the potatoes and chicken and then return the baking sheet to the oven.
4. Allow the potatoes and chicken to roast until the chicken has an internal temperature of Fahrenheit 165 degrees, about thirty-five to forty-five minutes. Remove the roasted yellow potatoes and chicken from the oven and allow it to rest for five minutes before serving.

Tex-Mex Chicken and Zucchini

This simple casserole is full of flavor! Perfect for when you are craving Tex-Mex, such as tacos or burritos. It contains your favorite aspects of Tex-Mex, but, but without the hassle or mess. Enjoy this casserole on its own, or top it with your favorite garnishes, such as guacamole or salsa verde. This casserole is also great served over cooked whole grains, such as brown rice.

The Servings: 6
The Time to Prepare/Cook: 30 minutes
The Calories: 347
The Ingredients:
Chicken breast, boneless and skinless, cut into 1" pieces – 1 pound
Onion, diced – 1
Bell peppers, diced – 2
Corn kernels – 1 cup
Zucchini, diced – 2
Diced tomatoes, canned – 14 ounces
Black beans, cooked – 1.75 cups
Cilantro, fresh, chopped – 0.5 cup
Green onions, chopped – 0.5 cup
Colby Jack cheese, shredded – 1 cup
Sea salt – 1 teaspoon
Cumin, ground – 1 tablespoon
Taco seasoning – 1 teaspoon
Black pepper, ground – 0.25 teaspoon
Garlic, minced – 5 cloves
Extra virgin olive oil – 1 tablespoon

The Instructions:
1. Warm a large skillet over medium-low and add in your bell pepper, onion, garlic, and olive oil. Allow the vegetables to sauté for three minutes, while occasionally stirring.
2. Ad your chopped chicken breast, black pepper, and sea salt to the skillet, sautéing for five minutes while again stirring every so often.
3. Into the skillet, add your zucchini, black beans, corn kernels, diced tomatoes, cumin, and taco seasoning. Continue stirring and cooking the skillet for ten minutes. The chicken should be fully cooked at this stage, with an internal temperature of Fahrenheit 165 degrees.
4. Sprinkle the Colby Jack over the top of the skillet and cook for just a few minutes, until the cheese has melted. Lastly, garnish with green onion and cilantro before serving.

Cuban Chicken and Rice

You will be shocked at how flavorful and healthy these bowls are, despite being incredibly easy and quick to make! With this recipe, you can have a full delicious meal in a matter of minutes, if you just keep a few ingredients in stock.

The Servings: 3
The Time to Prepare/Cook: 15 minutes
The Calories: 476
The Ingredients:
Chicken breast, boneless and skinless – 1 pound
Extra virgin olive oil – 1 tablespoon
Black beans, cooked – 0.33 cup
Brown rice, cooked – 1 cup
Sea salt – 0.5 teaspoon
Oregano, dried – 0.5 teaspoon
Cumin, ground – 1 teaspoon
Garlic, minced – 1 teaspoon
Black pepper, ground – 0.25 teaspoon
Pineapple, diced – 1 cup
Avocado, diced – 1
Tamari sauce or coconut aminos – 2 teaspoons
Orange, juiced – 1
Lime – 1, divided

The Instructions:
1. In a large skillet over medium-high, add the olive oil. Once the oil is hot and shimmering, add in the chicken breasts. Sprinkle the sea salt and pepper over the chicken, and sear each side of the breast for five to six minutes. The chicken is ready when they are nicely seared with an internal temperature of Fahrenheit 165 degrees. If your chicken breasts are more thick than usual, you might want to just slightly pound them with a meat mallet so that they are of average thickness.
2. Meanwhile, dice both the avocado and pineapple. Toss half of your lime juice with the diced avocado, to prevent browning.
3. Once the chicken breast pieces are done cooking, remove it from the skillet and allow it to rest for a few minutes.
4. Into the now empty skillet add the garlic, oregano, and cumin, allowing the spices to toast for one minute. Add in your tamari sauce, orange juice, and sea salt. Allow this sauce to simmer in the skillet until it has reduced by half.
5. Meanwhile, warm the rice and beans, tossing them together.
6. To create your bowls, divide all of the ingredients into thirds to create three servings. First place the rice and beans in the bottom of your bowls, followed by the pineapple, avocado, chicken, and lastly the mojo sauce. Garnish the bowls with the remaining half of the lime.

Cheesy Meatballs

These meatballs are tender, flavorful, and cheesy—they will simply melt in your mouth! Enjoy them with your choice of sides, such as whole grains, pasta, zucchini noodles, or spaghetti squash. You can even make a meatball sandwich with homemade bread! However you choose to serve these meatballs, you are sure to love them.

The Servings: 8
The Time to Prepare/Cook: 35 minutes
The Calories: 300
The Ingredients:
Ground turkey – 2 pounds
Egg – 1
Parmesan, shredded – 0.5 cup
Mozzarella, shredded – 1 cu
Black pepper, ground – 0.5 teaspoon
Red pepper flakes – 0.5 teaspoon
Italian herb blend – 0.5 teaspoon
Onion powder – 2 teaspoons
Garlic, minced – 2 teaspoons
Sea salt – 1 teaspoon
Marinara sauce – 1 cup
Provolone, shredded – 1 cup

The Instructions:
1. Warm your oven to Fahrenheit 400 degrees and grease a casserole dish or medium-sized baking pan.
2. In a bowl, combine together your ground turkey with the garlic, herbs, spices, Parmesan, and mozzarella cheeses. You want to fully combine the meat and flavorings without overworking the meat, or it will get tough.
3. Use a small cookie scoop or regular spoon to create evenly sized meatballs, about two tablespoons in size each. Roll the portions into balls and then arrange them in your greased baking dish.
4. Place the baking dish in the oven, cooking for fifteen to twenty minutes, until the meatballs have an internal temperature of Fahrenheit 165 degrees. Remove the baking pan from the oven and drain off any excess grease.
5. Pour the marinara sauce of your choice over the top of the ground turkey meatballs and then sprinkle the provolone over the top of that. Return the turkey meatballs and cheese to the oven until the cheese is melted and bubbling, about seven minutes. Remove the meatballs with marinara and cheese from the oven and serve the meatballs with your choice of sides.

Fish Taco Bowls

Enjoy these bowls over your choice of whole grains, such as brown rice or buckwheat groats. You can also add your choice of other traditional fish taco toppings, such as red cabbage, coleslaw, or pineapple. However you choose to serve these bowls, you will love the fresh flavors of the corn salsa and avocado cream with the blackened fish!

The Servings: 6
The Time to Prepare/Cook: 30 minutes
The Calories: 322
The Fish Ingredients:
Tilapia fillets – 6
Black pepper, ground – 0.25 teaspoon
Oregano dried – 0.125 teaspoon
Smoked paprika – 0.5 teaspoon
Cumin, ground – 1 tablespoon
Chili powder – 1 tablespoon
Onion powder – 0.25 teaspoon
Cayenne pepper, ground – 0.25 teaspoon
Lime zest – 0.5 teaspoon
Garlic, minced – 4 cloves
Sea salt – 1 teaspoon
Extra virgin olive oil – 0.5 tablespoon
The Salsa Ingredients:
Corn kernels – 1 cup
Black beans, cooked – 1.5 cups
Red onion, diced – 0.66 cup
Jalapeno, diced – 1
The Avocado Cream Ingredients:
Sour cream, light – 1 cup
Avocado, diced – 1
Sea salt – 0.25 teaspoon
Lime zest – 0.5 teaspoon
Lime juice – 1 tablespoon
Cilantro, fresh, chopped – 0.25 cup
Black pepper, ground – 0.25 teaspoon
The Instructions:
1. In a small kitchen mixing dish, combine the onion powder, oregano, paprika, black pepper, cayenne, cumin, chili powder, and sea salt from the fish list of ingredients. Rub this blend over both sides of all of the fish fillets.
2. Warm a large skillet over medium-high with the extra virgin olive oil. Add in the garlic and allow it to sauté for half a minute. Add in two of your tilapia fillets and allow them to sear for two to three minutes, undisturbed.
3. Flip the fillets over and sear the second side for about two minutes. Once the fillets are fully cooked and opaque, transfer them to a separate dish and cook the remaining fillets in the same way. Top the cooked fillets with the lime zest.

4.   Meanwhile, prepare the corn salsa in a separate skillet. In this skillet combine the onion, jalapeno, and corn kernels. Allow them to cook over medium-high for a couple minutes without stirring, so that they can sear.
5.   After about two minutes, give them a stir and allow them to sear for another two minutes, until caramelized and tender. Stir in the cooked black beans and cook for another minute until warm, and then remove the salsa from the heat.
6.   Lastly, prepare the avocado cream by blending all of the ingredients together in a blender or food processor until creamy.
7.   To assemble your bowls, place any cooked grains you are using in the bottom of the bowl, followed by the corn salsa, tilapia, and lastly the avocado cream. Enjoy the bowls while warm and freshly made.

Cilantro Lime Salmon

Salmon is one of the best options when it comes to getting more healthy fats in your diet, as it is high in omega-3s! With this recipe, you can enjoy a delicious salmon fillet with whatever sides you choose to serve it with.

The Servings: 6
The Time to Prepare/Cook: 20 minutes
The Calories: 295
The Ingredients:
Salmon fillet – 1.5-2 pounds
Garlic, minced – 4 cloves
Lime juice – 2 tablespoons
Sea salt – 0.75 teaspoon
Extra virgin olive oil – 0.33 cup
Date paste – 3 tablespoons
Red pepper flakes – 0.5 teaspoon
Cilantro, fresh, chopped – 3 tablespoons
Black pepper, ground – 0.25 teaspoon
The Instructions:
1.   Warm your oven to Fahrenheit 350 degrees and line a large baking sheet with kitchen parchment or a silicone mat. Place your large salmon fillet on top of the prepared baking sheet and sprinkle the sea salt and black pepper over the top.
2.   In a bowl, whisk together the date paste, lime juice, olive oil, and red pepper flakes. Spread this mixture over your salmon before placing it in the oven. Allow it to bake until it is cooked through and flakes when poked with a fork, about fifteen to twenty minutes.
3.   The last five minutes of cooking your salmon fillet, turn your oven's broiler on to caramelize the cilantro lime glaze over the top of the salmon fillet. After removing your fish from the oven, sprinkle the cilantro over the top and serve.

Salmon Patties

These salmon patties are a great all-purpose entree that you can serve along with your favorite side dishes or in a bun as a sandwich with a bit of coleslaw. However you choose to serve these patties, you are sure to love them!

The Servings: 8
The Time to Prepare/Cook: 40 minutes
The Calories: 279
The Ingredients:
Salmon fillet – 1 pound
Black pepper, ground – 0.5 teaspoon
Garlic powder – 0.5 teaspoon
Sea salt – 0.75 teaspoon
Extra virgin olive oil – 5 tablespoons, divided
Onion, diced – 1 cup
Bell pepper, diced – 0.66 cup
Egg, lightly beaten – 2
Parsley, fresh, chopped – 0.25 cup
Breadcrumbs, whole-grain – 1 cup
Mayonnaise – 3 tablespoons
Worcestershire sauce or tamari sauce – 1 teaspoon

The Instructions:
1. Warm your oven to Fahrenheit 425 degrees and line a baking sheet with kitchen parchment and a silicone mat.
2. Place your salmon fillet on the baking sheet, with the skin facing downward. Brush one tablespoon of your olive oil over the top of the fish. Sprinkle the sea salt, garlic powder, and black pepper over the top. Place the fish in the oven until cooked through and flaky, about fifteen minutes.
3. Allow the baked salmon to rest for ten minutes. Once it has rested, use two forks to flake the meat, placing the meat in a bowl and discarding any bones and skin.
4. Meanwhile, in a large skillet over medium heat add two tablespoons of your oil along with the bell pepper and onion, sautéing them until tender, about seven to ten minutes. Remove the skillet of vegetables from the heat.
5. Add your sautéed onion and bell pepper into the bowl with your flaked salmon meat, along with the mayonnaise, Worcestershire or tamari sauce, breadcrumbs, beaten eggs, and parsley. Stir together to combine. Form the mixture into eight evenly sized patties, about two heaping tablespoons in size each. Use your hands to shape the patties so that they resemble a burger patty.
6. Into a large skillet, add your last two tablespoons of extra virgin olive oil and place several of your patties in the skillet. You don't want to overcrowd the salmon patties in the pan, so only place as many patties in the pan as can easily fit while still having a bit of space between them. Allow the patties to sear on both sides for three to four minutes, until golden, and then remove them from the pan to cook the remaining patties. When removing the patties from the skillet, place them on a plate with a clean kitchen towel, to remove any excess oil. Serve warm with your favorite condiments.

Turkey Meatloaf

This meatloaf is a comfort food classic! You will love how tender and delicious it is, despite being made with turkey. Enjoy it as a comforting dinner with your favorite sides or place the leftovers inside a sandwich for a killer lunch.

The Servings: 8
The Time to Prepare/Cook: 1 hour, 35 minutes
The Calories: 273
The Ingredients:
Ground turkey – 2 pounds
Zucchini, shredded – 2 cups
Eggs, beaten – 2
Breadcrumbs, whole-grain – 0.5 cup
Milk of choice – 0.25 cup
Italian herb seasoning – 1 teaspoon
Black pepper, ground – 1 teaspoon
Garlic powder – 2 teaspoons
Onion powder – 2 teaspoons
Worcestershire sauce or tamari sauce – 1 tablespoon
Sea salt – 1 teaspoon
Feta cheese – 1 cup
Marinara sauce – 1 cup, divided

The Instructions:
1. Warm your oven to Fahrenheit 350 degrees and line a large baking sheet with kitchen parchment or a silicone mat.
2. Prepare the zucchini by first shredding it and then placing in on the center of a clean kitchen towel. Bundle the edges of the towel up around the zucchini and then squeeze the wrapped zucchini to press as much of the natural liquid from the squash out as possible, leaving the zucchini somewhat dry. Set the zucchini aside.
3. In a large kitchen mixing dish, mix together the breadcrumbs and your choice of milks. Once it forms a paste, add in the zucchini, eggs, Worcestershire sauce, feta cheese, ground turkey, and half of the marinara sauce. Mix together the meatloaf until the ingredients are evenly distributed.
4. Transfer the meatloaf mixture onto your prepared baking pan, and use your hands to shape it into a nice loaf. Spread the remaining prepared marinara sauce of choice over the top of the meatloaf and then place the baking sheet in the oven.
5. Allow your meatloaf to bake until it has an internal temperature of Fahrenheit 165 degrees, about an hour and fifteen minutes. Remove the turkey meatloaf from the oven and allow it to rest for five minutes before slicing and serving.

Chicken with Caramelized Onions and Mushrooms

This chicken is full of flavor from the caramelized onions, mushrooms, and garlic, making it simply delicious! Enjoy this chicken with any of your favorite side dishes and you are sure to have a delicious meal that can impress anyone.

The Servings: 6
The Time to Prepare/Cook: 45 minutes
The Calories: 399
The Ingredients:
Chicken breasts, boneless skinless – 6, medium
Mushrooms, sliced – 8 ounces
Onions, thinly sliced – 2
Garlic, minced – 5 cloves
Sea salt – 1 teaspoon
Extra virgin olive oil – 2 tablespoons
Balsamic vinegar – 2 tablespoons
Chicken broth – 0.5 cup
Black pepper, ground – 0.5 teaspoon

The Instructions:
1. Add one tablespoon of your oil to a large oven-safe skillet and sear both sides of the chicken breasts for four minutes each over medium heat. Remove the boneless/skinless seared chicken breasts from the pan, and set it aside.
2. Add the remaining tablespoon (three teaspoons) of extra virgin olive oil to the pan along with the onions, and cook them over medium-low heat while occasionally stirring until they begin to caramelize—about fifteen minutes. You may need to reduce the heat of the oven-safe skillet a bit, so that they caramelize rather than burn.
3. Warm your oven to Fahrenheit 400 degrees.
4. Stir the mushrooms into the onions and cook for five more minutes, until the edges are browned. Mix in your chicken broth and balsamic vinegar.
5. Nestle the chicken breasts into the onions and mushrooms and place the skillet in the oven for ten to fifteen minutes, until the chicken is fully cooked with an internal temperature of Fahrenheit 165 degrees. Remove the pan of chicken, mushrooms, and onions from the oven and allow the chicken to rest for a few minutes before serving.

Chicken Parmesan Pasta Bake

This pasta bake is a classic that makes it easy to create a full and delicious meal in a single pan. You can easily assemble this meal with little effort, giving you a complete meal in less than an hour. You can even get creative with this pasta bake, adding in some of your favorite vegetables, if you would like.

The Servings: 6
The Time to Prepare/Cook: 45 minutes
The Calories: 483
The Ingredients:
Whole-grain pasta, uncooked – 1 pound
Chicken breast, boneless skinless – 1 pound
Marinara sauce – 3 cups
Tomatoes, diced, canned – 1.75 cups
Italian herb seasoning – 1 teaspoon
Sea salt – 1 teaspoon
Red pepper flakes – 0.5 teaspoon
Breadcrumbs, whole-grain – 0.5 cup
Parmesan cheese, shredded – 2 tablespoon
Mozzarella cheese, shredded – 1 cup

The Instructions:
1. Cook the whole-grain pasta in a large pot of boiling water until it is tender with still a little bite remaining, and then drain off the water. Meanwhile, warm the oven to Fahrenheit 400 degrees and chop the chicken into small bite-sized pieces.
2. In a nine-by-thirteen-inch baking pan, toss together the pieces of chicken with the cooked pasta, diced tomatoes, red pepper flakes, sea salt, and marinara sauce. Once well combined, cover the baking pan with kitchen aluminum and place it in the oven for thirty minutes.
3. In a small bowl, combine together the breadcrumbs with the Italian herb seasoning and the Parmesan cheese.
4. After the pasta has baked for thirty minutes, remove the aluminum covering. Sprinkle the shredded mozzarella cheese over Chicken Parmesan pasta bake followed by the breadcrumb mixture. Allow the dish to bake for ten to fifteen more minutes without the aluminum, until the mozzarella cheese has melted over the chicken pasta and turned golden in color. Remove the chicken Parmesan pasta bake from the oven and enjoy it hot.

Creamy Potato Soup

You will love this creamy and comforting potato soup! You will be surprised how creamy it can be, even if you choose to use dairy-free milk! For this recipe, I recommend avoiding coconut milk. However, dairy, almond, cashew, and soy milk are all great choices!

The Servings: 4
The Time to Prepare/Cook: 45 minutes
The Calories: 250
The Ingredients:
Potatoes, peeled and chopped – 1 pound
Celery, diced – 0.5 cup
Carrots, diced – 1 cup
Onion, diced – 1 cup
Vegetable broth – 4 cups
Milk of choice – 2 cups
Extra virgin olive oil – 2 tablespoons
Sea salt – 0.75 teaspoon
Garlic powder – 1 teaspoon
Rosemary, chopped – 1 teaspoon
Black pepper, ground – 0.5 teaspoon
The Instructions:
1. In a large pot, add the extra virgin olive oil, celery, onion, and carrots. Allow these vegetables to sauté together over medium until the onions turn translucent, usually about ten minutes.
2. Add all of the remaining ingredients for the creamy potato soup, except for the milk, to the pot and give it a good stir. Bring the creamy potato soup to a boil and then reduce it to a simmer, allowing it to simmer until the potatoes are fork-tender, about thirty minutes.
3. Remove the creamy potato soup from the heat and stir in your milk of choice. Using a stand blender or immersion blender, blend the pot of soup until completely smooth and creamy. If you are using a stand blender, you will probably have to blend it in two different batches.
4. Serve the soup immediately or warm it back up on the stove for a few minutes before serving.

White Bean Soup with Lemon

You will love the fresh and zesty flavor the lemon gives this soup, which pairs perfectly with the earthy herbs. This recipe uses canned white beans for a quick and easy soup, but you can also use home-cooked beans, if you would like. If you choose to go that route, then you will want to use five cups of white beans.

The Servings: 4
The Time to Prepare/Cook: 25 minutes
The Calories: 474
The Ingredients:
Onion, diced – 1
Celery, diced – 2 stalks
Garlic, minced – 2 cloves
Carrots, diced – 3
Extra virgin olive oil – 2 tablespoons
Tahini paste – 2 tablespoons
White beans, drained and rinsed – 3 cans
Vegetable broth – 4 cups
Lemons, juiced – 2
Sea salt – 0.5 teaspoon
Thyme, dried – 0.5 teaspoon
Rosemary, dried – 0.5 teaspoon
Black pepper, ground – 0.25 teaspoon

The Instructions:
1. In a large pot, sauté the celery, carrots, and onion in the extra virgin olive oil until tender, about seven minutes. Add in your herbs and garlic and sauté for one more minute, until fragrant.
2. Add your tahini paste, white beans, vegetable broth, and seasonings to the pot and stir it all together. Bring the white bean soup to a boil before reducing it to a simmer and allowing it to all meld together for ten minutes.
3. Remove the white bean soup from the heat, stir in the lemon juice, and serve the soup warm.

Roasted Tomato Soup

This roasted tomato soup is simply to die for! You will find it is much better than any canned variety you have ever tried. Enjoy this sandwich alone, or paired with a classic grilled cheese made with whole-grain bread and pure real cheese. For this recipe, I recommend avoiding coconut milk. However, dairy, almond, cashew, and soy milk are all great choices!

The Servings: 4
The Time to Prepare/Cook: 1 hour, 40 minutes
The Calories: 280
The Ingredients:
Roma tomatoes, sliced in half lengthwise – 9
Onion, diced – 1
Garlic, minced – 4 cloves
Extra virgin olive oil – 4 tablespoons, divided
Sea salt – 1 teaspoon
Basil, fresh, chopped – 1 cup
Thyme, fresh, chopped – 1 tablespoon
Black pepper, ground – 0.5 teaspoon
Date paste – 1 tablespoon
Vegetable broth – 2 cups
Milk of choice – 0.66 cup
San Marzano crushed tomatoes – 28 ounces

The Instructions:
1. Warm your oven to Fahrenheit 375 degrees. On a baking pan, toss together your sliced tomatoes with the black pepper, sea salt, and half of the olive oil. Place this pan in the oven and allow the tomatoes to roast for one hour.
2. In a large pot, add the remaining olive oil along with the onions, sautéing them for five minutes until lightly tender and then add in the minced garlic and chopped fresh thyme. Sauté for one more minute, until the herbs and garlic are fragrant.
3. Stir the date paste, basil leaves, and crushed tomatoes into your pot and allow them to simmer together for ten minutes. Stir in the roasted tomatoes and vegetable broth, allowing the soup to simmer for an additional thirty minutes. Be sure to stir your soup occasionally to prevent sticking and burning.
4. Use an immersion blender or stand blender to completely blend the soup until smooth. Once blended, stir in the milk of choice and then serve.

Green Enchilada Soup

If you enjoy enchiladas, then you will love this soup! It is creamy, cheesy, and full of salsa verde! You will find that not only is this soup delicious freshly made, but it is even better after being chilled for a day while the flavors meld together.

The Servings: 8
The Time to Prepare/Cook: 1 hour
The Calories: 375
The Ingredients:
Chicken breasts – 2.5 pounds
Chicken broth – 3 cups
Milk of choice – 1 cup
Salsa verde – 4 ounces
Green enchilada sauce – 28 ounces
Cream cheese, low-fat, at room temperature – 4 ounces
Monterey Jack cheese, shredded – 2 cups
Black pepper, ground – 0.25 teaspoon
Sea salt – 0.5 teaspoon

The Instructions:
1. In a large pot, add the chicken breast chicken and broth, simmering the two together until the chicken breast is fully cooked int he broth and can easily be torn apart. Remove the chicken from the pot and shred it with a couple of forks before returning it to the pot.
2. Into the pot with the chicken, add the milk, enchilada sauce, cream cheese, salsa verde, and Monterey Jack cheese. Stir the soup together while it warms until the cheeses have melted. Add in your seasonings, give the soup a taste, and adjust the seasonings to your preference. Serve the soup hot.

Minestrone Soup

This minestrone soup is an Italian classic! You will love how vibrant and robust it is, while being incredibly simple and quick to make. For the best meal, serve it with a little freshly grated Parmesan over the top and a slice of homemade bread.

The Servings: 4
The Time to Prepare/Cook: 45 minutes
The Calories: 147
The Ingredients:
Vegetable broth – 4 cups
Onion, diced – 0.33 cup
Celery, diced – 1 cup
Carrot, chopped – 1 cup
Garlic, minced – 2 cloves
Tomato paste – 3 tablespoons
Sea salt – 0.5 teaspoon
Basil, dried – 2 teaspoons
Thyme, dried – 0.75 teaspoon
Oregano, dried – 1 teaspoon
Bay leaf – 1
Black pepper, ground – 0.25 teaspoon
Tomatoes, diced – 32 ounces
White beans, cooked – 0.25 cup
Red beans, cooked – 0.25 cup
Zucchini, sliced – 1
Baby spinach – 1 cup
Whole-wheat or brown rice pasta, dried – 0.25 cup
Balsamic vinegar – 1 teaspoon
Water

The Instructions:
1. In a large pot, sauté together the olive oil with the celery, carrots, onions, and garlic. Sauté them in this way until the vegetables are slightly softened, about four minutes. Stir in the herbs and cook for one additional minute, until the herbs are fragrant.
2. Stir in the vegetable broth, tomato paste, diced tomatoes, and the cooked beans. Add just enough water to cover your vegetables. Bring the minestrone soup to a boil and then reduce it to a simmer, cooking for twenty minutes.
3. Stir in the zucchini and dried pasta and cook for an additional ten minutes, until your pasta is tender. Lastly, add in the spinach, balsamic vinegar, and seasonings, cooking until the spinach has wilted, about one minute. Remove the minestrone soup from the heat and serve warm.

Chicken Barley Soup

This soup is perfect for the autumn months, when you are feeling ill, or simply whenever you want a simple meal that is cozy and hearty. This soup is incredibly easy with only a few ingredients, making it incredibly easy to prepare, even if you are under the weather.

The Servings: 4
The Time to Prepare/Cook: 70 minutes
The Calories: 355
The Ingredients:
Chicken breast – 2
Chicken broth – 5 cups
Black pepper, ground – 0.25 teaspoon
Extra virgin olive oil – 1 tablespoon
Celery, diced – 2 stalks
Onion, diced – 0.5
Carrots, chopped – 3
Thyme, dried – 0.5 teaspoon
Rosemary, dried – 0.5 teaspoon
Sea salt – 0.5 teaspoon
Pearl barley – 0.66 cup

The Instructions:
1. In a large pot sauté your onions, celery, and carrots in the olive oil until the onions turn translucent, about five minutes. Stir in the barley, chicken broth, seasonings, and the whole chicken breasts.
2. Bring your soup to a simmer, cover with a lid, and allow it to cook until the chicken breast in the soup is cooked through and the barley is tender, about forty-five minutes to an hour. Be sure to give your chicken barley soup an occasional stir.
3. Remove the chicken breasts from the soup and shred it with a pair of forks. Stir it back into the chicken barley soup before serving.

Carrot Ginger Soup

This soup is full of heart-healthy and anti-inflammatory ingredients! Chicken soup has long been known as a cold remedy, but this soup is incredibly more powerful. It only takes thirty minutes to make, so even when you are really sick, you can quickly prepare some to get you feeling better. Of course, you can also keep some ready made in the freezer for those emergencies when you suddenly come down with a stomach bug or the flu.

The Servings: 4
The Time to Prepare/Cook: 35 minutes
The Calories: 363
The Ingredients:
Carrots, chopped – 5 cups
Ginger, peeled and grated – 2 tablespoons
Garlic, minced – 4 cloves
Onion, diced – 1
Extra virgin olive oil – 1 tablespoon
Vegetable broth – 4 cups
Lime, juiced – 0.5
Sea salt – 0.75 teaspoon
Thyme leaves, dried – 1 teaspoon
Black pepper, ground – 0.5 teaspoon
Coconut milk, full-fat – 13.5 ounces
The Instructions:
1. In a large pot, sauté the onion in the olive oil for five to six minutes, until tender. Stir in the garlic and ginger, cooking for an additional minute until fragrant.
2. Into the pot, stir the remaining herbs and seasonings along with the carrots and vegetable broth. Allow this to all simmer together until the carrots are tender, about twenty to thirty minutes.
3. Using a stand blender or an immersion blender, blend the carrot soup until smooth and creamy. Stir in the lime juice and coconut milk and then serve the soup warm.

Seafood Chowder

This chowder is perfect for seafood lovers, as it contains both shrimp and fish! Enjoy the soup alone or with a slice of your favorite homemade bread. Keep in mind, that this chowder should be served within two days of preparation, so that the seafood stays fresh.

The Servings: 6
The Time to Prepare/Cook: 30 minutes
The Calories: 412
The Ingredients:
Shrimp, peeled and cleaned – 2 pounds
Cod fillets, chopped into 1" pieces – 1.75 pound
Sea salt – 0.5 teaspoon
Garlic, minced – 2 cloves
Red pepper flakes – 1 teaspoon
Lime juice – 0.33 cup
Black pepper, ground – 0.5 teaspoon
Water – 3 tablespoons
Cornstarch – 2 tablespoons
Extra virgin olive oil – 2 tablespoons
Tomatoes, diced – 2
Onion, diced – 1
Bell pepper, diced – 2
Seafood broth – 0.5 cup
Cilantro, fresh, chopped – 0.5 cup
Coconut milk, full-fat – 1 cup

The Instructions:
1. Begin by marinating the shrimp and fish. To do this, stir them together in a bowl with the lime juice, sea salt, red pepper flakes, and black pepper. Cover the bowl and place it in the fridge while you sauté your vegetables.
2. In a large pot, sauté the onion in the olive oil until translucent, about four minutes. Stir in the bell peppers and sauté for two more minutes before stirring in the seafood broth. Allow the broth to warm with the vegetables for a minute or two.
3. Add the bowl containing the seafood and marinade into the pot along with the diced tomatoes. Simmer the chowder until the shrimp and fish are opaque and cooked through, about ten minutes. Be sure to gently stir it occasionally.
4. In a small bowl, whisk together the cornstarch and water to form a slurry. Stir the slurry into the soup pot and continue simmering the chowder for one minute before removing it from the heat. Lastly, stir in the cilantro and coconut milk before serving.

Creamy Asparagus Soup

This soup is creamy, light, and delicious! Enjoy it alone or paired together with your favorite sandwich or salad. It is also great with a little fresh Parmesan grated over the top.

The Servings: 4
The Time to Prepare/Cook: 30 minutes
The Calories: 228
The Ingredients:
Cannellini beans, cooked – 1.75 cups
Asparagus, trimmed and chopped – 2 pounds
Onion, diced – 1
Garlic, minced – 2 cloves
Extra virgin olive oil – 1 tablespoon
Vegetable broth – 4 cups
Lemon zest – 0.25 teaspoon
Black pepper, ground – 0.25 teaspoon
Lemon juice – 1 tablespoon
Sea salt – 0.5 teaspoon
The Instructions:
1. In a large pot, sauté the onion in the olive oil until it is translucent, about five minutes. Add in the garlic, asparagus, cannellini beans, black pepper, and sea salt, sautéing for two more minutes.
2. Pour the vegetable broth into the pot and bring it to a boil before reducing it to a simmer and cooking until the asparagus is tender, about five minutes. Remove the soup from the heat.
3. Using a stand blender or immersion blender, blend the soup until it is completely smooth and creamy. Stir in the lemon zest and lemon juice and then serve while warm.

Classic Reuben

This classic sandwich is ideal for pumpernickel bread, as the deep dark flavor pairs wonderfully with the contents. This sandwich is especially perfect for people who love the bright zesty and zingy flavors of corned beef and sauerkraut. Keep in mind that prepared sandwich meats from the store should be avoided, as they are pro-inflammatory. Instead, prepare your own sandwich meats.

The Servings: 1
The Time to Prepare/Cook: 5 minutes
The Calories: 597
The Ingredients:
Pumpernickel bread – 2 slices
Swiss cheese – 1 slice
Corned beef, thinly sliced – 4 ounces
Sauerkraut, drained and warmed – 0.25 cup
Thousand Island dressing – 2 tablespoons
The Instructions:
1. While you prepare your sandwich, warm a small skillet over medium heat.
2. Spread your thousand island dressing on one half of each slice of pumpernickel bread. On top of one of the slices spread in the dressing, layer your corned beef, Swiss cheese, and sauerkraut. Top this off with the remaining slice of pumpernickel bread. Of course, you want to layer this sandwich so that the thousand island dressing halves of the bread are facing inward, not outward.
3. Grease your warmed skillet and place your prepared sandwich inside it, flipping it once the first size is toasted until the second side matches. You might need to lower the pan heat if it is too hot, so that your bread doesn't burn before the cheese melts.
4. Remove the sandwich from the heat, slice it in half, and enjoy alone or with your favorite pickles.

Vegetable Medley Sandwich

This sandwich is full of warm roasted vegetables that perfectly complement the fresh tomatoes, alfalfa sprouts, and hummus. This sandwich is simply irresistible! Plus, if you use dairy-free pesto, this sandwich is even vegan.

The Servings: 4
The Time to Prepare/Cook: 40 minutes
The Calories: 334
The Roasted Ingredients:
Eggplant, sliced – 1
Zucchini, sliced – 1
Bell pepper, sliced – 1
Onion, sliced – 0.5
Sea salt – 0.5 teaspoon
Garlic powder – 1 teaspoon
Extra virgin olive oil – 2 teaspoons
Black pepper, ground – 0.25 teaspoon
The Sandwich Ingredients:
Bread – 8 slice
Alfalfa sprouts – 1 cup
Tomatoes, sliced – 2
Lettuce, chopped – 1 head
Pesto – 0.25 cup
Hummus – 0.5 cup
The Instructions:
1. Warm your oven to Fahrenheit 425 degrees and line a baking sheet with kitchen parchment or aluminum. Alternatively, you could simply grease the pan, though this will require a little extra cleanup.
2. In a bowl, toss together all of your vegetables, seasonings, and olive oil from the roasted ingredients list. Once the vegetables are evenly coasted, spread them onto the prepared baking sheet and allow them to roast until tender and browned, about thirty to thirty-five minutes.
3. To prepare your sandwich spread the hummus on one slice of your bread and then layer your roasted vegetables on top. Add your lettuce, tomatoes, and alfalfa sprouts. Spread your hummus on your other slice of bread, and then stack it on top of the stacked ingredients. Slice your sandwich in half before serving. Do this process for all four sandwiches. Alternately, you could make one sandwich now and save the remaining ingredients for quick sandwiches later on.

Cob Sandwich

This delicious cob sandwich contains roasted chicken, boiled eggs, avocado, and the other delicious ingredients you love from cob salad! For the best sandwich, try using the mayonnaise and bread recipes from this book.

The Servings: 1
The Time to Prepare/Cook: 5 minutes
The Calories: 602
The Ingredients:
Bread, sliced – 2
Lettuce – 2 leaves
Cheddar cheese – 1 slice
Tomato – 2 slices
Hard-boiled egg, sliced – 1
Roasted chicken, sliced – 2 ounces
Avocado, sliced – 0.25
Mayonnaise – 1 tablespoon
The Instructions:
1. Spread the mayonnaise on one half of each slice of the bread and then stack the lettuce, roasted chicken, cheddar cheese, boiled egg, tomato, and avocado on one of the slices. Place the other slice of bread over the top, slice your sandwich, and then serve.

Chick n' Sandwich

This sandwich gets its name not from chicken, but from chickpeas! These health legumes are great for your health and make a delicious alternative to chicken and egg salad. You can use either home-cooked or canned chickpeas when making this sandwich.

The Servings: 2
The Time to Prepare/Cook: 5 minutes
The Calories: 508
The Ingredients:
Chickpeas, cooked – 1.75 cups or one can
Mayonnaise – 2 tablespoons
Red onion, minced – 0.25 cup
Celery, minced – 0.33 cup
Pickles, minced – 0.33 cup
Garlic powder – 0.5 teaspoon
Black pepper, ground – 0.25 teaspoon
Lettuce – 2 leaves
Bread – 4 slices

The Instructions:
1. If you are using canned chickpeas, drain off all the liquid and give them a good rinse before using. Add your chickpeas to a bowl and mash them with a large fork or potato masher. You want them pretty broken down, but with still a bit of texture left. There might be a couple whole chickpeas here and there, which is okay.
2. Add the mayonnaise, ted onion, celery, pickles, garlic powder, and black pepper to your bowl and stir it together into the chickpeas until it is uniformly combined. Taste the chickpea salad and adjust the seasonings to your preference.
3. To prepare your sandwiches, top two slices of bread with half of the chickpea salad each. Top the mixture off with a lettuce leaf and another slice of bread. Slice both sandwiches in half before serving.

Hawaiian Chicken Sandwich

This sandwich uses barbecue sauce and Ranch dressing. For these, you want to use a healthy versions without sugar and pro-inflammatory additives. For delicious and easy barbecue sauce and Ranch that meet all the requirements of the anti-inflammatory diet, check out my other book, The Anti-Inflammatory Diet Action Plan.

The Servings: 4
The Time to Prepare/Cook: 30 minutes
The Calories: 470
The Ingredients:
Chicken breasts, raw and sliced – 1 pound
Coleslaw mix – 3 cups
Pineapple – 4 slices
Red onion – 4 slices
Ranch dressing – 0.25 cup
Barbecue sauce – 0.25 cup
Rice wine vinegar – 1 tablespoon
Butter lettuce – 8 leaves
Bread – 8 slices

The Instructions:
1. Warm your oven to Fahrenheit 425 degrees and an oven-safe skillet on the stove to medium-high. Once the skillet is warm, grease it and then add the sliced chicken breast. Sear the slices on each side, about four minutes total. Transfer the skillet to the oven, allowing the chicken to roast for an about ten minutes—until the internal temperature reaches Fahrenheit 165 degrees.
2. Meanwhile, pan-fry the pineapple slices in a skillet or even on a grill, until tender and warm.
3. Prepare the coleslaw by adding the coleslaw mix, Ranch dressing, and rice wine vinegar to a bowl, and tossing them all together.
4. To prepare your sandwiches, lay out the prepared coleslaw, pineapple, roasted chicken, and remaining ingredients in front of you. Toss the chicken in the barbecue sauce.
5. Lay out four slices of the bread and divide the barbecue chicken between them, laying the chicken on the top of each slice. Follow it up with the warm pineapple, coleslaw, red onion, and the lettuce. Stack your remaining four slices of bread over the top, slice the sandwiches in half, and then serve them.

Caprese Panini

This caprese panini contains all the elements of a caprese salad, but all deliciously grilled together inside your favorite bread. Don't worry if you don't have a panini press, as this sandwich can be prepared on the stove!

The Servings: 1
The Time to Prepare/Cook: 10 minutes
The Calories: 532
The Sandwich Ingredients:
Bread – 2 slices
Extra virgin olive oil – 1 tablespoon
Tomato, sliced – 1
Pesto – 1 tablespoon
Mozzarella cheese – 2 slices
The Glaze Ingredients:
Balsamic vinegar – 0.25 cup
Date paste – 0.25 teaspoon
The Instructions:
1.   Begin to prepare the glaze by adding the balsamic vinegar and date paste to a small saucepan. Place the saucepan over medium to medium-low heat until it has reduced to half (2 tablespoons). When doing this, be sure to not boil the glaze, you never want it to exceed a light simmer. Remove the pan from the heat and allow the glaze to cool.
2.   Using a pastry brush, lightly coat both sides of your bread slices with the olive oil. Place your bread in a skillet and grill the first side over medium on your stove until it is toasted.
3.   Flip both sides of your bread over and then on one slice of bread layer your pesto, mozzarella cheese, and sliced tomato. Drizzle a little bit of your balsamic glaze over this and then place your remaining slice of bread over the top, grilled-side-down.
4.   Once the first side of your sandwich has toasted, flip it over and allow the other side to toast until golden and your cheese is slightly melted. Remove the sandwich from the heat, slice it in half, and enjoy.

Spicy Tuna Wrap

These spicy tuna wraps uses sriracha, but feel free to try it out with any of your favorite healthy hot sauces. You could also make this into a sandwich rather than a wrap, if you would like.

The Servings: 2
The Time to Prepare/Cook: 5 minutes
The Calories: 340
The Ingredients:
Tuna, drained – 1 can
Onion, diced – 0.25 cup
Celery, diced – 0.25 cup
Sriracha hot sauce – 2 tablespoons
Mayonnaise – 2 tablespoons
Tomato, sliced – 1
Baby spinach – 0.33 cup
Whole-wheat tortillas – 2
The Instructions:
1. In a bowl, combine together your drained tuna, mayonnaise, sriracha, celery, and onion.
2. Divide the prepared tuna salad into two portions, placing each portion in the center of one of your tortillas. Top it with the baby spinach and tomato before tightly rolling up your wraps. Serve them whole or first slice them in half.

Side Dishes

Multi-Grain Pilaf with Mushrooms

This pilaf is a delicious and simple pilaf made with wheat berries and brown rice. But, even if you are allergic to gluten, you can still enjoy a version of this pilaf. For those with wheat allergies, simply replace the cooked wheat berries with an equal amount of cooked buckwheat groats or other whole grains. While this pilaf contains red wine, if you prefer, you could replace the wine with equal parts broth.

The Servings: 6
The Time to Prepare/Cook: 40 minutes
The Calories: 191
The Ingredients:
Wheat berries, cooked – 1.5 cups
Brown rice, cooked – 1.5 cups
Chicken broth – 0.25 cup
Red wine – 0.25 cup
Onion, diced – 1.5 cups
Mushrooms, sliced – 1 pound
Garlic, minced – 5 cloves
Extra virgin olive oil – 2 tablespoons
Sea salt – 0.75 teaspoon
Tamari sauce or coconut aminos – 1 tablespoon
Rosemary, fresh, chopped – 1 teaspoon
Thyme, fresh, chopped – 0.5 teaspoon
Lemon zest – 1 teaspoon
Black pepper, ground – 0.25 teaspoon

The Instructions:
1. In a large skillet over medium heat, sauté the onions, half of the sea salt, and the olive oil. Allow the onions to sauté until sweet and soft, about seven minutes. Add in the garlic and cook for one more minute, until fragrant.
2. Add the mushrooms and tamari sauce to the skillet cook for five more minutes, until the mushrooms are tender. Once soft, add in the chicken broth and red wine, simmering for five more minutes.
3. Stir the remaining sea salt into the skillet long with the herbs, lemon zest, and whole grains. Simmer for a few more minutes, until the liquid has been absorbed and evaporated, and then serve warm.

Herb-Scented Rice

This is a great all-purpose side dish to go alongside nearly any main dish. You will love the fresh bursting flavors! While this is a great rice dish, you can also try replacing the rice with any of your other favorite cooked whole grains, if desired.

The Servings: 4
The Time to Prepare/Cook: 10 minutes
The Calories: 236
The Ingredients:
Brown rice, cooked – 2 cups
Onion – 0.25 cup
Black pepper, ground – 0.25 teaspoon
Extra virgin olive oil – 0.25 cup
Parsley, fresh, chopped – 0.25 cup
Basil, fresh, chopped – 1 tablespoon
Thyme, fresh, chopped – 1 tablespoon
Garlic, minced – 3 cloves
Sea salt – 0.5 teaspoon
The Instructions:
1. Either chop and mince the onion, garlic, and herbs with a knife, or you can easily pulse them all in your food processor. Once all of the ingredients are minced, stir them together with the rice.
2. Warm the rice mixture either in a skillet or in the microwave, and serve either warm or at room temperature.

Toasted Rice with Mushrooms and Thyme

Rice doesn't have to be plain and boring. You can imbue it with delicious and rich flavors of fresh herbs, mushrooms, and extra virgin olive oil. Not only that, but by changing how you prepare it and choosing to toast it, you can give it a delicious nutty flavor.

The Servings: 6
The Time to Prepare/Cook: 50 minutes
The Calories: 148
The Ingredients:
Brown rice, uncooked – 1 cup
Garlic, minced – 4 cloves
Onion, diced – 0.5
Extra virgin olive oil – 1.5 teaspoons
Water – 1 cup
Vegetable broth – 1 cup
Cremini mushrooms, sliced – 8 ounces
Sea salt – 0.5 teaspoon
Thyme, fresh, chopped – 1 tablespoon
Parsley, fresh, chopped – 3 tablespoons
Black pepper, ground – 0.25 teaspoon

The Instructions:
1. Add half a teaspoon of your extra virgin olive oil and onion to a large saucepan and allow it to cook until tender, about five minutes over medium heat. Add in the garlic, stirring it until fragrant, about one minute.
2. Stir your rice into the saucepan, allowing it to toast for about one minute, until it smells nutty. Be careful not to burn the rice and keep stirring it. Once toasted, add in the water and vegetable broth, bringing the liquid to a boil before reducing it to a low simmer.
3. Cover the saucepan with a lid and allow it to simmer until the liquid has been absorbed by the rice, about thirty-five minutes.
4. Meanwhile, in a skillet, add the remaining olive oil and mushrooms to a skillet. Allow the mushrooms to sauté over medium-high until they are browned, about five minutes. Add in the thyme and toast for an added half minute. Remove the mushrooms from the heat.
5. Once the rice is cooked, stir it together with the sautéed mushrooms and remaining seasonings. Enjoy while warm with your favorite entree.

Spanish Cauliflower Rice

If you want to enjoy a low-calorie and low-carb side dish reminiscent of grains, then you will love this Spanish cauliflower rice! The cauliflower is "riced" by pulsing it in a food processor, creating tiny grain-like pieces. You can easily create this cauliflower rice yourself, or you can purchase it already riced and frozen, if you would like.

The Servings: 4
The Time to Prepare/Cook: 25 minutes
The Calories: 97
The Ingredients:
Cauliflower, riced – 4 cups
Sea salt – 1 teaspoon
Tomato paste – 3 tablespoons
Garlic, minced – 3 cloves
Jalapeno, minced – 1
Onion, minced – 1
Extra virgin olive oil – 1 tablespoon
Cumin – 1 teaspoon
Paprika – 0.5 teaspoon
Lime juice – 1 tablespoon
Cilantro, fresh, chopped – 3 tablespoons
Black pepper, ground – 0.25 teaspoon

The Instructions:
1. If you are ricing the cauliflower yourself, cut it into large chunks that are small enough to fit into your food processor. Have your device fitted with the S-blade and run the cauliflower through until it is all riced. You may need to empty the food processor bowl partway through, if the cauliflower fills it up. Alternatively, you can choose to buy cauliflower rice already prepared and frozen.
2. Warm a large skillet over medium and sauté your onions in the extra virgin olive oil until they become transparent, about five minutes. Add in the garlic and jalapeno, sautéing for an additional minute until fragrant.
3. Stir the black pepper, paprika, cumin, sea salt, and the tomato paste into the vegetables. Once combined, stir in your riced cauliflower. Sauté the cauliflower while occasionally stirring, so that it is fully combined with the vegetables and seasonings. Allow it to sauté until it has released and evaporated its liquid, creating tender and fluffy "rice."
4. Remove the cauliflower rice from the stove and top it with the lime juice and cilantro before serving.

Parmesan Roasted Green Beans

These green beans may be simple, but that allows them to truly shine! You will love the combination of Parmesan cheese, lemon, and toasted breadcrumbs that adorn the fresh green beans. Enjoy these beans best warm and fresh from the oven with any of your favorite entrees.

The Servings: 4
The Time to Prepare/Cook: 25 minutes
The Calories: 119
The Ingredients:
Green beans, fresh – 1 pound
Extra virgin olive oil – 2 tablespoons
Sea salt – 0.5 teaspoon
Lemon zest – 0.25 teaspoon
Garlic powder – 0.25 teaspoon
Parmesan cheese, grated – 2 tablespoons
Breadcrumbs, whole-grain – 2 tablespoons
The Instructions:
1. Warm your oven to Fahrenheit 400 degrees and prepare a large baking sheet.
2. In a kitchen mixing dish, toss the fresh green beans with all of the other ingredients, until they are fully coated. Spread the entire mixture from the mixing dish out onto your prepared baking sheet and place it in the oven.
3. Allow your beans to cook until they are tender and the breadcrumbs are toasted, about fifteen to twenty minutes. Halfway through the cooking time, give the green beans and breadcrumbs a good stir to promote even cooking. Remove the pan from the oven and enjoy!

Rosemary Sweet Potato Bites

These sweet potato bites have an inedible umami flavor from the natural sweetness of the potato, woodiness from the rosemary, and the depth of the Parmesan cheese. They are simply incredible! I love to keep these prepared and in the fridge at all times, so that I can always have a good go-to prepared side dish or snack.

The Servings: 6
The Time to Prepare/Cook: 40 minutes
The Calories: 189
The Ingredients:
Sweet potatoes, peeled and cut into 1" cubes – 2 pounds
Black pepper, ground – 0.5 teaspoon
Garlic powder – 0.5 teaspoon
Rosemary, fresh, chopped – 1 tablespoon
Sea salt – 1 teaspoon
Extra virgin olive oil – 2 tablespoons
Parmesan cheese, grated – 0.25 cup
The Instructions:
1. Warm your oven to Fahrenheit 425 degrees and prepare a large baking sheet.
2. Place your cubed sweet potatoes directly onto the baking sheet along with all of the ingredients except for the Parmesan cheese. Toss them all together, so that the potatoes are evenly coated in the oil and seasonings. Spread the potatoes out on the pan, so that they are in a single layer and bake evenly.
3. Place the baking sheet in the middle of your warm oven and bake the sweet potatoes until they are tender, about twenty to thirty minutes. Remove the baking pan from the oven and sprinkle the Parmesan evenly over the top of the sweet potatoes. Allow the potatoes to rest for five minutes while the Parmesan melts before serving.

Corn and Zucchini with Parmesan

This dish can be made year-round in most placed, as it is easy to find frozen corn and zucchini in the produce department. However, you will find it tastes the best during the summer months, when both corn and zucchini are at their peak. If possible, during these months, use the freshest corn and zucchini you can find for the best results.

The Servings: 4
The Time to Prepare/Cook: 15 minutes
The Calories: 138
The Ingredients:
Zucchini, diced – 1
Corn kernels – 1.75 cups
Garlic, minced – 4 cloves
Parmesan cheese, grated – 2 tablespoons
Lime juice – 2 tablespoons
Sea salt – 0.5 teaspoon
Basil, dried – 0.25 teaspoon
Thyme, dried – 0.25 teaspoon
Oregano, dried – 0.25
Black pepper, ground – 0.5 teaspoon
Extra virgin olive oil – 2 tablespoons
Parsley, fresh, chopped – 2 tablespoons
The Instructions:
1.   In a large skillet, sauté the garlic in the oil for one minute over medium heat until it becomes fragrant.
2.   Add the remaining ingredients except for the Parmesan and cilantro to the skillet with the toasted garlic and mix them together to combine. Allow the vegetables to cook through until tender, about eight to ten minutes.
3.   Remove the skillet from the heat and top it off with the Parmesan and cilantro before serving.

Garlic Roasted Broccoli

This broccoli is one of the simplest recipes in this book—but it is amazing! Many people don't like broccoli simply because of how it has been prepared for them. They have never tasted broccoli truly prepared correctly, until now. Try this recipe and you are sure to find a new appreciation for this staple vegetable.

The Servings: 4
The Time to Prepare/Cook: 25 minutes
The Calories: 125
The Ingredients:
Broccoli florets – 1.5 pound
Black pepper, ground – 0.25 teaspoon
Extra virgin olive oil – 2 tablespoons
Garlic, minced – 6 cloves
Sea salt – 0.5 teaspoon
The Instructions:
1. Warm your oven to Fahrenheit 450 degrees and prepare a large baking sheet.
2. Add your broccoli to your baking dish, drizzling the oil over the top followed by the garlic and seasonings. Toss all of this together, until the broccoli is evenly coated, and then smooth it out into an even layer on the baking sheet.
3. Allow the broccoli to roast until tender with browned edges, about twenty minutes. Remove from the oven and serve warm.

Golden Mashed Potatoes

These mashed potatoes are deceptively creamy and rich, you won't believe how healthy they are! While you could certainly prepare this recipe with russet or any other type of potato, it simply won't be the same. The Yukon gold potatoes make all the difference, as they contain an irresistible buttery flavor.

The Servings: 5
The Time to Prepare/Cook: 30 minutes
The Calories: 225
The Ingredients:
Yukon gold potatoes, peeled and quartered – 2 pounds
Sea salt – 1 teaspoon
Vegetable broth – 0.5 cup
Sour cream, light – 0.5 cup
Garlic, minced – 5 cloves
Extra virgin olive oil – 2 tablespoons
Black pepper, ground – 0.25 teaspoon
Chives, chopped – 3 tablespoons
The Instructions:
1. Bring a large pot of salted water to a boil, and then add in your quartered potatoes. Allow the potatoes to cook until they are fork-tender, about fifteen to twenty minutes.
2. Drain off the water from the cooked potatoes, leaving the potatoes in the pot. Into the pot, add your vegetable broth, olive oil, light sour cream, black pepper, garlic, and sea salt. Use a potato masher to mash the potatoes together with the other ingredients until it is smooth and creamy. Resist the urge to over mash the potatoes, as that will result in a more starchy potato. Taste the potatoes and adjust the salt level to your preference.
3. Serve the potatoes with the chives over the top and your choice of gravy.

Vibrant Slaw

This slaw is full of vibrant colors from the red and green cabbage, carrots, cilantro, and jalapeno. Not only does this give the slaw gorgeous color, but it gives it a bounty of anti-inflammatory nutrients and antioxidants. This is all dressed in an incredibly flavorful dressing, which perfectly accentuates the best flavors that the slaw has to offer.

The Servings: 8
The Time to Prepare/Cook: 20 minutes
The Calories: 147
The Slaw Ingredients:
Green cabbage, shredded – 3 cups
Red cabbage, shredded – 3 cups
Green onion, chopped – 0.5 cup
Cilantro, fresh, chopped – 1 cup
Carrots, shredded – 2 cups
Jalapeno, minced – 1
Almonds, sliced and toasted – 0.25 cup
Pepitas – 0.5 cup
The Dressing Ingredients:
Apple cider vinegar – 2 tablespoons
Extra virgin olive oil – 3 tablespoons
Sea salt – 0.5 teaspoon
Garlic, minced – 2 cloves
Date paste – 1 tablespoon
Cayenne pepper – 0.25 teaspoon (optional)
Black pepper, ground – 0.25 teaspoon
The Instructions:
1. In a large kitchen mixing dish, toss together all of the slaw ingredients, except for the pepitas and sliced almonds.
2. In a separate kitchen mixing dish, whisk together all of the dressing ingredients until combined and the date paste as fully incorporated. Pour your vibrant slaw dressing over the slaw and toss it all together until the slaw is evenly coated. Give the slaw a taste, and adjust the seasonings to your preference.
3. Place the slaw in the fridge to marinate with the dressing for at least an hour, or up to a full day.
4. When you are ready to serve the vibrant slaw, add the sliced almonds and pepitas and give it another good toss.

Chinese Chicken Salad

This Chinese chicken salad is the perfect addition to any East Asian meal. Whether you are serving a traditional Chinese meal or an anti-inflammatory dish prepared in the method of Chinese take-out, this salad is the perfect compliment. The tamari sauce, sesame, ginger, and garlic in this salad are the ideal compliments to your meal.

The Servings: 6
The Time to Prepare/Cook: 20 minutes
The Calories: 223
The Salad Ingredients:
Chicken, shredded – 2 cups
Red cabbage, shredded – 2 cups
Romaine lettuce, shredded – 3 cups
Carrots, shredded – 1 cup
Green onions, chopped – 0.5 cup
Cilantro, fresh, chopped – 0.5 cup
Almonds, slivered – 0.5 cup
Sesame seeds – 2 tablespoons
The Dressing Ingredients:
Tamari sauce or coconut aminos – 3 tablespoons
Sesame seed oil – 1 tablespoon
Ginger, peeled and grated – 1 tablespoon
Garlic, minced – 4 cloves
Rice wine vinegar – 3 tablespoons
Soybean oil – 1 tablespoon
Date paste – 2 teaspoons
Sea salt – 1 teaspoon
The Instructions:
1. In a large salad mixing dish, toss together all of the salad ingredients, except for the almonds and sesame seeds.
2. In a separate kitchen mixing dish, whisk together the dressing ingredients until fully combined. Pour half of the Chinese chicken salad dressing over the salad, give it a toss, and taste. You can add more Chinese dressing if you would like, or you can stop here. By only adding in a portion of the dressing at a time, you can more easily customize the flavor to fit your preferences.
3. Top the salad off with your almonds and sesame seeds before serving.

Roasted Brussels Sprouts Kale Salad

If you want a salad that will truly impress, then you must try this one! The warm roasted Brussels sprouts perfectly pair with the fresh kale and apple, which are then dressed with a simple but flavorful dressing. This salad is perfect for autumn, when the kale, apple, and Brussels sprouts are all in season.

The Servings: 6
The Time to Prepare/Cook: 30 minutes
The Calories: 234
The Salad Ingredients:
Kale, ribs removed and chopped – 4 cups
Apple, diced – 2
Green onions, chopped – 0.5 cup
Cranberries, dried – 0.33 cup
The Brussels Sprouts Ingredients:
Brussels sprouts, sliced in half – 1 pound
Black pepper, ground – 0.125 teaspoon
Extra virgin olive oil – 3 tablespoons
Garlic, peeled – 5 cloves
Sea salt – 0.125 teaspoon
Parmesan cheese, grated – 0.5 cup
The Dressing Ingredients:
Extra virgin olive oil – 1 tablespoon
Sea salt – 0.5 teaspoon
Lemon juice – 1 tablespoon
Mayonnaise – 2 tablespoon
Dijon mustard – 1 tablespoon
Date paste – 1 tablespoon
Black pepper, ground – 0.25 teaspoon
The Instructions:
1. Warm your oven to Fahrenheit 400 degrees and prepare a large oven-safe skillet. You can use a stainless-steel skillet, but cast iron is ideal. Warm the skillet on the stove over medium heat.
2. Add the Brussels sprouts, olive oil, and garlic to the warm skillet. Arrange the sprouts so that the cut side is facing downward to caramelize. Sprinkle the sea salt and black pepper over the top.
3. Allow the Brussels sprouts to sear and caramelize for a couple minutes. Once seared, give the sprouts a good stir with a spatula and transfer the skillet to the hot oven. Allow the sprouts to roast until tender, about ten minutes. Stir them halfway into their cooking time. About one minute before removing the sprouts from the oven, sprinkle the Parmesan over the top so that it can melt.
4. Meanwhile, prepare the salad. To do this, toss together the kale apple, green onion, and cranberries in a large salad kitchen dish. In a separate small kitchen mixing dish, whisk together the dressing ingredients until combined. Add the prepared simple dressing to the Brussels sprouts and kale salad and toss it all together.
5. Top the prepared salad with the warm Brussels sprouts before serving.

Mediterranean Quinoa Salad

With this salad, you will feel as if you are right at home in your favorite Greek restaurant! The fresh vegetables combined with the pickled olives and soft feta cheese and garnished with an olive oil vinaigrette is irresistible.

The Servings: 6
The Time to Prepare/Cook: 20 minutes
The Calories: 357
The Ingredients:
Quinoa, uncooked – 1 cup
Water – 1.5 cups
Avocado, diced – 2
Bell pepper, diced – 1
Cucumber, diced – 1
Tomato, diced – 1
Red onion, minced – 0.25 cup
Cilantro, fresh, chopped – 0.5 cup
Kalamata olives, pitted – 1 cup
Feta cheese, crumbled – 0.5 cup
Sea salt – 0.5 teaspoon
Cumin, ground – 1 tablespoon
Lemon juice – 3 tablespoons
Extra virgin olive oil – 3 tablespoons
Black pepper, ground – 0.25 teaspoon

The Instructions:
1. Add your uncooked quinoa and water to a saucepan, bringing it to a boil. Cover the pot with a lid and reduce the heat to low, allowing it to simmer for twelve minutes. Remove the now cooked quinoa pan from the heat and allow the quinoa to rest for five minutes before removing the lid from the quinoa and fluffing it with a fork.
2. Add all of your ingredients, including the cooked quinoa, to a mixing dish and toss it all together until it is evenly combined and coated. Taste the salad and adjust the seasoning to your preferences before serving.

Southwestern Salad

This Southwestern salad is full of flavor and essential nutrients! The corn, black beans, lettuce, and other vegetables are all perfectly accented with a creamy and delicious avocado cilantro dressing that you won't soon forget! But, if you are someone who doesn't care for cilantro, feel free to replace it with parsley instead.

The Servings: 5
The Time to Prepare/Cook: 15 minutes
The Calories: 316
The Salad Ingredients:
Bell pepper, diced – 1
Grape tomatoes, sliced in half – 10 ounces
Black beans, cooked – 1.75 cup
Green onions, chopped – 0.5 cup
Corn kernels, cooked – 2 cups
Romaine lettuce, chopped – 1 head
The Dressing Ingredients:
Garlic, minced – 3 cloves
Lime juice – 2 tablespoons
Sea salt – 0.25 teaspoon
Cumin, ground – 0.5 teaspoon
Avocado – 0.5
Cilantro, fresh, chopped – 1 cup
Extra virgin olive oil – 0.25 cup
Date paste – 2 teaspoons
White wine vinegar – 1.5 teaspoons
The Instructions:
1. In your blender or food processor, combine together all of the dressing ingredients until smooth and creamy. Give the southwestern salad dressing a taste and adjust the seasoning to your preference.
2. In a large kitchen mixing dish, toss together all of the southwestern salad ingredients. Add the southwestern dressing and toss again to coat, and then serve immediately.

Autumn Apple Salad

This salad is incredibly simple, yet incredibly flavorful. The mixed greens pair beautifully with the fruit, nuts, and blue cheese, all of which is then dressed in a sweet and zesty dressing. To make this salad ahead of time, simply prepare both of the salad and dressing components separately and wait to toss the two together directly before eating.

The Servings: 6
The Time to Prepare/Cook: 10 minutes
The Calories: 333
The Salad Ingredients:
Mixed greens – 6 cups
Pear, diced – 1
Apple, diced – 1
Cranberries, dried – 0.33 cup
Pecans, toasted – 0.5 cup
Blue cheese – 0.5 cup
The Dressing Ingredients:
Extra virgin olive oil – 0.5 cup
Sea salt – 1 teaspoon
Date paste – 2 tablespoon
Dijon mustard -1 teaspoon
Lime juice – 0.25 cup
Black pepper, ground – 0.5 teaspoon
The Instructions:
1. In a large salad mixing dish, toss together all of the salad components.
2. In a separate kitchen mixing dish, whisk together the dressing ingredients.
3. Directly before serving your salad, add the prepared dressing, tossing the two together.

Tender Carrot Slaw

This tender carrot slaw is great as a side dish to any of your favorite entrees, but it can also make a good snack or meal in itself. Create a sandwich with your favorite bread and this slaw as the filling, and you are really in for a treat!

The Servings: 2
The Time to Prepare/Cook: 5 minutes
The Calories: 228
The Ingredients:
Carrots, grated – 1 pound
Sea salt – 0.5 teaspoon
Extra virgin olive oil – 2 tablespoons
Apple cider vinegar – 2 tablespoons
Garlic, minced – 2 cloves
Red onion, minced – 0.25 cup
Parsley, fresh, chopped – 2 tablespoons
Cilantro, fresh, chopped – 2 tablespoons
Black pepper, ground – 0.25 teaspoon

The Instructions:
1. Grate the carrots for the tender slaw either in a food processor or with a box grater and then add them to a kitchen mixing dish along with the remaining slaw ingredients. Toss all of them together, until the carrots are fully and evenly coated. Give the slaw a taste and adjust the seasonings to your preference.
2. You can serve the slaw immediately or you can allow it to marinade for five minutes to an hour first. The longer you marinade the slaw, the better it will taste.

Appetizers and Snacks

Cheesy Quinoa Bites

These cheesy bites are quick and easy to make for a delicious snack! To make them as quickly as possible for last-minute snacks, I recommend keeping some pre-cooked quinoa and vegetables in the fridge. Keeping these hands will not only be great for this recipe, but for easy meals, as well.

The Servings: 4
The Time to Prepare/Cook: 30 minutes
The Calories: 220
The Ingredients:
Quinoa, cooked – 1 cup
Egg, beaten – 1
Sea salt – 0.5 teaspoon
Cheddar cheese, shredded – 1 cup
Broccoli, steamed, chopped – 0.5 cup
Carrots, steamed, chopped – 0.5 cup
Onion, minced – 0.25 cup
Garlic, minced – 2 cloves
Black pepper, ground – 0.25 teaspoon

The Instructions:
1. Warm your oven to Fahrenheit 350 degrees and grease a mini muffin tin.
2. In a mixing dish, toss together all of your ingredients until fully combined. You want to make sure that for these quinoa bites the egg, cheese and seasonings are easily distributed.
3. Divide the quinoa mixture between all of the greased cups in your mini muffin tin, pressing the mixture down to firmly compact it. Place the pan in the middle of your oven and allow it to bake until crispy and golden-brown in color, about fifteen to twenty minutes.
4. Allow the bites to cool for five minutes before removing them from the oven.

Bruschetta

This bruschetta is delicious when you use homemade whole-grain bread, such as the recipes from this book! Use whatever type of bread you like, as long as it is a healthy whole-food variety. Even if you use grain-free bread, like some of the recipes in this book, that's okay as long as it is made with healthy anti-inflammatory ingredients.

The Servings: 5
The Time to Prepare/Cook: 20 minutes
The Calories: 194
The Ingredients:
Bread, whole-grain – 10 slices
Extra virgin olive oil – 4 teaspoons, divided
Sea salt – 0.25 teaspoon
Garlic, minced – 2 cloves
Balsamic vinegar – 1 tablespoon
Basil, fresh, chopped – 0.33 cup
Parmesan, grated – 0.25 cup
Roma tomatoes, seeded and diced – 8
Black pepper, ground – 0.25 teaspoon

The Instructions:
1. In a mixing dish, prepare the topping for your bruschetta by combining the tomatoes, Parmesan, basil, garlic, sea salt, balsamic, one teaspoon of olive oil, and black pepper. Once combined, cover the kitchen mixing dish and place it in the fridge to marinate while you move onto the next step.
2. Heat a grill pan for the bruschetta over medium heat on your stovetop, or you can use a gas grill to medium heat or a charcoal grill until the coals have paled in color.
3. While your grill heats, slice each slice of bread in half, so that you are left with twenty small pieces rather than ten large ones. Using a pastry brush, use the remaining tablespoon of olive oil to brush over the bread slices on both sides.
4. Grill both sides of the bruschetta bread until toasted with visible grill marks and then remove it, adding your chilled brochette toppings and serving immediately.

Cashew Chicken Lettuce Wraps

These lettuce wraps are just like something you would find at a high-end Chinese restaurant. You will love the depth of flavor of the cashews combining with the delicious sauce and chicken. You can easily make the chicken filling ahead of time, storing it until you are ready for a snack.

The Servings: 6
The Time to Prepare/Cook: 20 minutes
The Calories: 345
The Ingredients:
Chicken breast, boneless skinless, cut into 1" pieces – 2 pounds
Extra virgin olive oil – 4 teaspoons
Tamari sauce or coconut aminos – 0.33 cup
Black pepper, ground – 0.25 teaspoon
Chicken broth – 0.75 cup
Garlic, minced – 2 teaspoons
Cashews, raw – 0.75 cup
Cornstarch – 2 tablespoons
Sea salt – 0.5 teaspoon
Sesame seed oil – 0.5 teaspoon
Sriracha sauce – 1 teaspoon
Date paste – 2 teaspoons
Rice vinegar – 1.5 tablespoons
Chinese five spice blend – 0.25 teaspoon
Butter lettuce – 2 heads

The Instructions:
1. In a large skillet over medium heat, add your extra virgin olive oil and your chicken. Sprinkle the sea salt and black pepper over the chicken, giving it a stir and spreading the chicken out into a single layer so that it can evenly cook. Allow the first side of the chicken to sear for three minutes before giving it a stir and continuing to cook until all sides of the chicken are golden-brown and fully cooked through. The cooked chicken breast should have an internal temperature of Fahrenheit 165 degrees.
2. Reduce the heat of the stove to low and stir in the garlic, allowing it to cook for another couple of minutes until the garlic has become fragrant.
3. Meanwhile, whisk together all of the remaining ingredients, except for the lettuce, in order to create your cashew sauce. Stir this mixture into your skillet once the garlic has toasted, and stir it allowing it to simmer until the cashew sauce thickens and coats the chicken.
4. Remove the chicken and cashew sauce mixture from the heat and serve it with the lettuce as wraps. To do this, simply add a little chicken mixture into the center of a leaf of lettuce, and enjoy!

Smoked Salmon Tea Sandwiches

These tea sandwiches are delicious classic, especially when you use homemade whole-grain bread, such as the recipes from this book! Use whatever type of bread you like, as long as it is a healthy whole-food variety. Even if you use grain-free bread, like some of the recipes in this book, that's okay as long as it is made with healthy anti-inflammatory ingredients.

The Servings: 6
The Time to Prepare/Cook: 20 minutes
The Calories: 213
The Ingredients:
Bread, whole-grain – 6 slices
Cream cheese, softened – 7 ounces
Sour cream, light – 2 tablespoons
Smoked salmon – 8 ounces
Dill, fresh, chopped – 2 tablespoons
Sea salt – 0.5 teaspoon
The Instructions:
1.   Start by slicing your bread slices (of average size) in half so that you are left with twelve small slices rather than six large ones.
2.   In a kitchen mixing dish, combine together your sour cream, cream cheese, dill, and sea salt until combined. Divide this mixture between your twelve slices of bread, spreading it over the top of each slice of bread. Then, top each slice with your smoked salmon.
3.   You can serve the sandwiches immediately, or chill them until ready to serve. Enjoy as open-faced sandwiches.

Creamy Cucumber Dill Bites

These bites only take a few minutes to whip up, but offer a great snack or an easy appetizer that you can share. Whether you need a snack for yourself in the middle of the workday or are looking to something to serve to company, you will find these an easy, fresh, and flavorful option.

The Servings: 6
The Time to Prepare/Cook: 10 minutes
The Calories: 171
The Ingredients:
English cucumber – 4
Grape tomatoes – 2 cups
Dill, fresh, chopped – 3 tablespoons
Cream cheese, softened – 8 ounces
Greek yogurt, plain – 0.5 cup
Sea salt – 0.5 teaspoon
Parsley, fresh, chopped – 2 tablespoons
Onion powder – 0.5 teaspoon
Garlic powder – 0.5 teaspoon
Black pepper, ground – 0.25 teaspoon
The Instructions:
1.   Slice your English cucumbers into rounds, about one-half inch thick. You can choose to either peel them or not, or even only partially peel them for an appealing striped look. Choose whichever method you prefer! Slice the grape tomatoes in half lengthwise.
2.   In a kitchen mixing dish, combine together the cream cheese, Greek yogurt, dill, sea salt, parsley, onion powder, garlic powder, and black pepper. This is easiest done with a hand beater, so that the seasonings are evenly distributed.
3.   Transfer the cream cheese mixture into a large plastic bag or a piping bag and cut off one tip of a bottom corner, to turn it into a piping bag. Hold the bag in both hands and pipe the mixture onto your cucumber rounds, and then top them off with the tomato halves.
4.   You can serve these bites immediately or chill them first.

Garlic Chili Edamame

These edamame only take a few ingredients that are really simple to keep on hand, especially since edamame is often sold frozen! This means that you can keep it stored in the freezer, without worrying about it spoiling, therefore allowing you to have an accessible snack any time of the year.

The Servings: 4
The Time to Prepare/Cook: 15 minutes
The Calories: 222
The Ingredients:
Edamame – 1 pound
Sesame seed oil – 0.5 teaspoon
Extra virgin olive oil – 2 tablespoons
Garlic, minced – 3 cloves
Chili paste – 2 tablespoons
Date paste – 1 teaspoon
Sea salt – 1 teaspoon
The Instructions:
1. Head a large skillet over medium-high heat and wait for it to warm up before adding in your edamame. Allow your edamame to sear undisturbed until the bottom sides are charred, and then give them a light stir. Let the pods cook this way, until both sides are charred and tender. Remove the edamame from the skillet and set it aside.
2. Reduce the heat of the stove to medium and then add in the garlic, allowing it to toast for about thirty seconds. Add in the remaining ingredients, stirring together until combined, and then add back in the charred edamame. Cook the edamame in the sauce for a minute or two before removing it from the heat and serving warm.

Mini Avocado Hummus Quesadillas

These mini quesadillas are incredibly simple but absolutely delicious! I like to always keep some hummus prepared in the fridge, so that I always have it on hand for dishes such as this one. If you are allergic to avocado, feel free to replace it with steamed or roasted vegetables of your choice.

The Servings: 4
The Time to Prepare/Cook: 15 minutes
The Calories: 227
The Ingredients:
Tortillas, whole-wheat – 4
Cilantro, fresh, chopped – 1 tablespoon
Cumin, ground – 0.25 teaspoon
Hummus – 0.25 cup
Queso fresco, crumbled – 1.5 ounces
Avocado, sliced – 0.5
The Instructions:
1. In a kitchen mixing dish, stir together the hummus, cilantro, and cumin. Spread this seasoned hummus mixture over one side of each tortilla. Divide the avocado and queso between the tortillas, layering it on one half of the side with the hummus. Fold the half with nothing but hummus over the avocado and cheese half, so that the avocado is nestled between a top and bottom layer of both tortilla and hummus.
2. Warm your skillet over medium heat and then add in two of your folded quesadillas, cooking each side for two to three minutes. After the first two have cooked, remove them from the skillet and cook the remaining two servings. Remove the quesadillas from the heat and serve warm.

Deviled Eggs

Deviled eggs are a great protein-rich snack full of flavor! Feel free to adjust the seasonings and garnishes to your taste, as long as you use anti-inflammatory ingredients. Also, keep in mind that it's important to use high-quality ingredients when making these—you don't want to use a mayonnaise full of pro-inflammatory additives. Instead, use the recipe for mayonnaise from this book.

The Servings: 4
The Time to Prepare/Cook: 30 minutes
The Calories: 178
The Ingredients:
Eggs – 6
Mayonnaise – 6 tablespoons
Dijon mustard – 2 teaspoons
Sea salt – 0.5 teaspoon
Paprika, smoked – 0.25 teaspoon
Black pepper, ground – 0.25 teaspoon
The Instructions:
1. Add your eggs to a large pot of cold water and place it on the stove. Bring the water the eggs are into a boil before reducing it to a simmer, allowing it to simmer for seven minutes. Remove the pot of water and boiled eggs from the heat, drain off the water, and place the eggs in a mixing dish of ice water to chill for a few minutes.
2. Peel the eggs and rinse any tidbits of shells off of them. Slice the eggs in half lengthwise and then carefully remove the egg yolk with a spoon, adding the yolk to a mixing dish and placing the egg whites onto a plate, setting them aside.
3. Use a fork to break apart the egg yolks, pressing them into small pieces before adding in the remaining ingredients. Stir together the mixture until it is well-combined and then give it a taste, adjusting the seasoning to your liking. Using a spoon, stuff the egg whites with the yolk mixture where the yolk had originally been until they are all stuffed. Serve immediately, or you can chill until you like.

Sweet and Spicy Cauliflower

This cauliflower is extremely low in calories, making it a great option for when you are looking to lose weight but still need a snack to tide you through the afternoon. While this dish is best enjoyed fresh from the oven, you can still prepare it ahead of time if you need a snack you can simply chill and reheat later for an instant energy boost.

The Servings: 4
The Time to Prepare/Cook: 35 minutes
The Calories: 110
The Cauliflower Ingredients:
Cauliflower florets – 4 cups
Black pepper, ground – 0.25 teaspoon
Sesame seed oil – 1 tablespoon
Garlic powder – 0.5 teaspoon
Sea salt – 0.5 teaspoon
Green onion, chopped – 1 tablespoon
The Sauce Ingredients:
Cornstarch – 1 teaspoon
Sriracha – 4 teaspoons
Date paste – 0.25 cup
Tamari sauce or coconut aminos – 5 tablespoons
Garlic, minced – 3 cloves
Onion powder – 0.5 teaspoon
Chinese five spice powder – 0.25 teaspoon
The Instructions:
1. Warm your oven to Fahrenheit 400 degrees and line a baking sheet with kitchen parchment or a silicone mat.
2. Add the cauliflower florets to your prepared baking sheet, spreading them out and then greasing them with cooking spray or brushing the extra virgin olive oil. Sprinkle your seasonings for the sweet and spicy cauliflower over the florets, tossing until evenly coated.
3. Place the spiced cauliflower florets in the oven until the edges of the cauliflower crowns, about fifteen to twenty minutes.
4. Meanwhile, combine all of the sweet and spicy sauce ingredients in a saucepan, cooking them over medium heat until bubbly and thickened.
5. After you remove your roasted cauliflower florets from the oven, allow them to rest for a couple of minutes before tossing the roasted florets in the prepared sweet and spicy sauce. Serve the sweet and spicy cauliflower while hot.

Breads

Whole-Wheat Sandwich Bread

This is the perfect bread for all your sandwich needs! It's nice and light and fluffy. The milk adds richness, which you will love, and you will also appreciate that you can use whatever type of milk you prefer. Want cows milk? That's great! Soy milk? That works, too! Almond milk? Sure, why not? This makes it a great option for people with allergies, as you can easily customize it to fit your needs.

The Servings: 12
The Time to Prepare/Cook: 3 hours, 20 minutes
The Calories: 190
The Ingredients:
White whole-wheat flour – 3.5 cups
Extra virgin olive oil – 0.25 cup
Date paste – 0.25 cup
Milk of choice, warm – 1.125 cup
Sea salt – 1.25 teaspoon
Active dried yeast – 2.5 teaspoons

The Instructions:
1. Prepare a nine-by-five inch loaf pan by lining it with kitchen parchment and then lightly greasing it.
2. In a large kitchen mixing dish, mix together all of your ingredients with a spatula. Once combined, leave the contents to rest for thirty minutes.
3. Begin to knead your dough until it is soft, stretchy, and pliable—about seven minutes. You can do this kneading by hand, but using a stand mixer and dough hook is the easiest method.
4. With the kneaded dough in its previously used mixing dish, cover the mixing dish with kitchen plastic or a clean damp kitchen towel in a warm location to rise until doubled in size, about an hour or two.
5. Gently, punch down your dough and shape it into a nice log before placing it in your prepared loaf pan. Cover the pan with the previously used plastic or towel and allow it to rise in the warm space until it has doubled in size, another hour or two.
6. When the bread is nearly done rising, warm your oven to Fahrenheit 350 degrees.
7. Remove the covering from your risen bread loaf and set the loaf in the middle of your hot oven. Carefully place aluminum foil over the loaf without deflating it, to prevent it from browning too quickly. Allow the bread to cook in this way for thirty-five to forty minutes before removing the foil and continuing to bake the bread for twenty minutes. The bread is ready when it is a gorgeous golden color and sounds hollow when you knock on it.
8. Allow the whole-wheat sandwich bread to cool in the pan for five minutes before removing it from the metal and transferring it to a wire rack to finish cooling. Allow the bread to cool completely before slicing.

Pumpernickel Bread

This classic bread is full of a deep and rich flavor that you will love! Enjoy it best with rustic sandwich toppings or soups. It is delicious, even if you only top it with a little of your favorite butter or cheese. You won't regret making yourself a pumpernickel sandwich for any meal.

The Servings: 12
The Time to Prepare/Cook: 2 hours, 30 minutes
The Calories: 221
The Ingredients:

Pumpernickel flour – 3 cups
Whole-wheat flour – 1 cup
Cornmeal – 0.5 cup
Cocoa powder – 1 tablespoon
Active dried yeast – 1 tablespoon
Caraway seeds – 2 teaspoons
Sea salt – 1.5 teaspoons
Water, warm – 1.5 cups, divided
Date paste – 0.25 cup, divided
Avocado oil – 1 tablespoon
Sweet potatoes, mashed – 1 cup
Egg wash – 1 egg white + 1 tablespoon water

The Instructions:
1. Prepare a nine-by-five inch loaf pan by lining it with kitchen parchment and then lightly greasing it.
2. In a saucepan, combine one cup of your water along with the cornmeal until it is hot and thick, about five minutes. Be sure to continue stirring while it heats to prevent lumps. Once thick, remove the pan from the heat and stir in your date paste, cocoa powder, caraway seeds, and avocado oil. Set the pan aside until the contents are cooled to lukewarm.
3. Add your remaining one-half cup of warm water into a large kitchen mixing dish along with the yeast, stirring it until the yeast has dissolved. Allow this mixture for the pumpernickel bread to sit for about ten minutes until it has bloomed and formed puffy bubbles. This is best done in a warm location.
4. Once the yeast has bloomed, add the lukewarm cornmeal water mixture into the mixing dish, along with the mashed sweet potatoes. Once the liquids and potato are combined, stir in the whole-wheat and pumpernickel flours. Knead the mixture for ten minutes, preferably with a stand mixer and dough hook. The dough is ready when it forms a cohesive ball that is smooth and pulls away from the edges of the mixing dish.
5. Remove the dough hook and cover your mixing dish with kitchen plastic or a clean damp kitchen towel. Place the kitchen mixing dish in a warm location to rise until the dough has doubled in size—about one hour.
6. Warm your oven to Fahrenheit 375 degrees in preparation for the bread loaf.
7. Shape the dough into a nice log shape and place it in your prepared loaf pan. Whisk together your egg wash and then use a pastry brush to lightly brush it over the top of your prepared loaf. If desired, use a sharp knife to score the loaf for a decorative design.
8. Place your loaf in the middle of your hot oven and allow it to bake until it is a gorgeous dark color and when you knock on it produces a hollow-like sound—about one hour. Remove the pumpernickel bread loaf from the oven and allow it to cool in the pan for five minutes before removing the pumpernickel bread from the pan and transferring the loaf to a wire rack to continue cooling. Don't slice the loaf until it is completely cool.

Gluten-Free Sandwich Bread

This sandwich bread is perfect not only for sandwiches, but also for any other recipe that may call for bread—whether it is toast or bread pudding. For best results, store this bread in the fridge once it's completely cool with a paper towel to absorb any moisture. When making this bread, keep in mind that potato starch is different from potato flour.

The Servings: 12
The Time to Prepare/Cook: 3 hours, 30 minutes
The Calories: 115
The Ingredients:
Buckwheat flour – 1 cup
Potato starch – 0.75 cup
Brown rice flour – 0.5 cup, plus 2 tablespoons
Psyllium husk – 0.25 cup
Sea salt – 2 teaspoons
Apple cider vinegar – 2.5 teaspoons
Water, warm – 1.66 cup, divided
Date paste – 2 tablespoons
Active dried yeast – 2.5 teaspoons

The Instructions:
1. Prepare a nine-by-five inch loaf pan by lining it with kitchen parchment and then lightly greasing it.
2. In a mixing dish, whisk together two-thirds of a cup of the warm water, date paste, and yeast until the contents are fully dissolved. Allow this mixture to sit for five to ten minutes, until the yeast has bubbled and puffed up—this should be done in a warm environment.
3. In a small mixing dish, whisk together the remaining cup of warm water with the psyllium husk and allow it to sit for half a minute to form a gel.
4. In the mixing dish of a stand mixer, combine the brown rice flour, buckwheat flour, potato starch, and sea salt. Once the yeast has bloomed, add it to the mixing dish along with the prepared psyllium gel and the apple cider vinegar.
5. Use the dough hook on your stand mixer to knead the dough on medium-low speed until the gluten-free sandwich dough is smooth and begins to form a ball that pulls away from the edges of the mixing dish—about five to ten minutes.
6. Once done kneading, cover the mixing dish with kitchen plastic or a clean damp kitchen cloth and allow the gluten-free dough to rise in a warm space until doubled in size, about one hour.
7. After the gluten-free sandwich dough has risen punch it down and form it into a nice loaf inside of the prepared loaf pan. Cover the pan with the leftover cloth or plastic and allow it to sit in a warm place to rise until doubled, another hour.
8. Meanwhile, warm the oven to Fahrenheit 475 degrees. While the oven warms, place a pan with a few inches of hot water in it in the bottom of the oven to create steam.
9. Once the bread loaf has risen, use a sharp knife and cut three straight scores down the middle of the loaf. Place the gluten-free sandwich loaf in the center of the

oven, above the pan of steaming water. Allow the bread to cook in the steam of the oven for twenty minutes without opening the door or being disturbed in any way. You don't want the steam to escape the oven.

10. After the initial twenty minutes have passed, remove the tray of water from the oven. Allow the oven to cook for an additional forty-five minutes without the steam. The gluten-free sandwich bread is done when it is a deep brown and sounds hollow when you knock on it.

11. Remove the pan of gluten-free bread from the oven and allow the bread to cool for five minutes before removing the loaf from the pan. Transfer the gluten-free sandwich loaf to a wire rack and allow it to cool completely before slicing.

Quinoa Protein Bread

This bread is perfect for when you need a boost of protein, one of the body's essential nutrients. From a single serving of this delicious whole-grain and gluten-free bread, you can get seven grams of protein. For even more protein, enjoy it with your favorite meats, cheeses, or nut butters.

The Servings: 12
The Time to Prepare/Cook: 1 hour, 45 minutes
The Calories: 233
The Ingredients:

Chickpea flour – 1 cup
Toasted quinoa flour – 1 cup
Potato starch – 1 cup
Sorghum flour – 1 cup
Xanthan gum – 2 teaspoons
Sea salt – 1 teaspoon
Water, warm – 1.5 cups

Active dry yeast – 1.5 teaspoons
Date paste – 2 tablespoons
Poppy seeds – 1 tablespoon
Sunflower seeds – 1 tablespoons
Pepitas – 2 tablespoons
Avocado oil – 3 tablespoons
Eggs, room temperature – 3

The Instructions:

1. Prepare a nine-by-five inch loaf pan by lining it with kitchen parchment and then lightly greasing it.
2. In a kitchen mixing dish, whisk together the warm water, date paste, and yeast until the contents are fully dissolved. Allow this mixture for the quinoa bread to sit for five to ten minutes, until the yeast has bubbled and puffed up—this should be done in a warm environment.
3. Meanwhile, in a larger mixing dish, preferably for a stand mixer, combine together the flours, starch, xanthan gum, and sea salt until combined. Lastly, in a small mixing dish, whisk together the avocado oil and eggs. Set these aside while you wait for the yeast to finish blooming.
4. Once the yeast has bloomed, turn the stand mixer with the flour mixture on low and pour in the yeast mixture. Allow the stand mixer with the paddle attachment to combine the liquid and flour for a few moments before adding in the egg and oil mixture. Continue allowing this mixture to combine for two minutes until it forms a cohesive dough ball. Add the seeds into the dough and mix for one more minute on medium speed. Keep in mind that the dough will be wetter and less elastic than dough made with traditional flour, as it is gluten-free.
5. Pour the quinoa protein dough into the prepared pan, cover it with kitchen plastic or a clean damp rag, and allow it to rise in a warm location free of drafts until doubled in size—about forty minutes. Meanwhile, warm the oven to Fahrenheit 375 degrees.
6. Place the risen loaf in the middle of your oven and allow it to bake until cooked through and golden-brown in color. When you knock on the quinoa protein bread loaf it should sound hollow. Remove the quinoa protein bread pan from the oven and allow it to cool for five minutes before removing the quinoa protein bread from the baking pan and transferring it to a wire rack to finish cooling. Allow the quinoa bread loaf to cool completely before slicing.

Zucchini Bread

This bread is sweet and full of flavor, you will be surprised how healthy it is! Without refined flour or sugars, it still retains the texture you crave from the fresh grated zucchini and applesauce. Enjoy this zucchini bread liberally as a snack, side dish, breakfast, or even dessert.

The Servings: 6
The Time to Prepare/Cook: 70 minutes
The Calories: 170
The Ingredients:
White whole-wheat flour – 2 cups
Baking soda – 1 teaspoon
Baking powder – 2 teaspoons
Sea salt – 0.5 teaspoons
Cinnamon, ground – 2 teaspoons
Egg, large – 1
Vanilla extract – 1 teaspoon
Applesauce, unsweetened – 0.5 cup
Zucchini, grated – 2 cups
Lakanto monk fruit sweetener – 0.75 cup

The Instructions:
1. Warm the oven to Fahrenheit 350 degrees and line a nine-by-five inch loaf pan with kitchen parchment or grease it.
2. In a large kitchen mixing dish, whisk together the applesauce, zucchini, vanilla extract, monk fruit sweetener, egg, and vanilla extract. In a separate mixing dish, combine the dry ingredients so that you don't get any lumps from the baking powder or soda.
3. Add the mixed dry ingredients for the zucchini bread into the wet ingredients and gently fold the two together, just until combined. Scrape the mixing dish clean, pouring the contents into the prepared loaf pan.
4. Place your zucchini bread loaf in the oven and allow it to bake until cooked completely through. It is ready when once inserted a toothpick can be removed cleanly—about one hour.
5. Remove the zucchini bread pan from the oven and allow it to cool for ten minutes before removing the zucchini bread loaf from the pan and transferring the loaf to a wire rack to finish cooling. Wait for the zucchini loaf to cool completely before slicing it.

Whole-Grain Cornbread

This corn bread is the perfect comfort food side dish. Enjoy it alone, with your favorite butter, or even with a little bit of date paste over the top. However you choose to serve this cornbread, whether as a side dish or even as a quick breakfast, you are sure to love it!

The Servings: 8
The Time to Prepare/Cook: 35 minutes
The Calories: 207
The Ingredients:
Yellow whole-grain cornmeal – 1 cup
White whole-wheat flour -1 cup
Egg – 1
Date paste – 2 tablespoons
Extra virgin olive oil – 0.33 cup
Sea salt – 1 teaspoon
Baking powder – 1 tablespoon
Baking soda – 0.5 teaspoon
Almond milk – 1 cup

The Instructions:
1. Warm the oven to Fahrenheit 400 degrees and prepare an eight-inch round baking dish or cast iron pan for the bread. Liberally grease the pan.
2. In a mixing dish, whisk together the cornmeal, whole-wheat flour, sea salt, and leavening agents until combined.
3. In a separate kitchen mixing dish, whisk together the remaining ingredients just until combined. Add in the flour mixture, folding the two together just until combined.
4. Pour the cornbread batter into the prepared pan and place it in the oven until golden-brown and fully set in the center, about twenty-five minutes. Remove the cornbread from the oven and allow it to cool for five minutes before slicing.

Sauces, Gravies, and Marinades

Date Paste

This paste is a great sweetener option! Many of the recipes in this book call for a bit of date paste when a recipe needs just a small amount of sweetness. But, remember, this should only be used in moderation. While dates are a healthier form of sugar—they are still sugar. This means that excessive amounts may increase inflammation. Everything in moderation, including this sweetener. If you need a larger amount of sweetener, I suggest stevia, monk fruit or erythritol.

The Servings: 20
The Time to Prepare/Cook: 5 minutes
The Calories: 80
The Ingredients:
Medjool dates, pitted – 24
Water, warm – 1 cup
The Instructions:
1. If your medjool dates are hard and dry, soak them in the warm water for an hour or two prior to making the paste. Or, you could soak them in boiling water for ten minutes. This won't be needed if your dates are fresh and soft.
2. Add the warm water and dates to your blender and blend until it forms a completely smooth paste without any chunks. When smooth, transfer it to an airtight container and store in the fridge for up to two weeks.

Cashew Queso Sauce

Whether you choose to eat cheese on the anti-inflammatory diet or not is a personal choice. While some people have absolutely no problem with dairy, there are many that do have sensitivities to dairy without even realizing it. If you are a person with these sensitivities, dairy can increase your inflammation. Thankfully, this is a delicious queso "cheese" sauce that anyone can enjoy—whether they eat dairy or not.

The Servings: 10
The Time to Prepare/Cook: 10 minutes
The Calories: 198
The Ingredients:
Water – 0.5 cup
Cashews, raw – 2 cups
Sea salt – 2 teaspoons
Lemon juice – 0.25 cup
Nutritional yeast – 0.5 cup
Rotel canned tomatoes with chilies – 28 ounces
Cilantro, fresh, chopped – 0.25 cup (optional)

The Instructions:
1. Start by soaking your cashews. To do this, you can simply pour some boiling water over them and allowing them to soak in them for five to fifteen minutes. You can also choose to boil them in a small saucepan of water.
2. Drain the boiled water off of your cashews and transfer the nuts to a blender. Into the blender, drain the liquid of the Ro-Tel tomatoes, adding only the liquid and not the tomatoes themselves yet at this point. Also add in the half cup of water, nutritional yeast, lemon juice, and sea salt. Allow this mixture to blend on high speed until it is completely smooth and creamy.
3. Pour the queso mixture from the blender and into a saucepan along with the tomatoes and chilies from the can. Allow this to gently warm up over medium-low until hot. Be careful to continue stirring and watching this closely, as the mixture can easily stick and burn. You can adjust the liquid level by adding more water if you want a thinner queso.
4. Remove the queso from the heat and stir in the cilantro, if you are using. Enjoy the queso hot!

Chimichurri Sauce

This classic chimichurri is incredibly fresh and delicious. You will love the versatility of this dish and all you can use it for. Try it as a marinade, a salad dressing, a garnish, or a dipping sauce. This seriously tastes good on almost any savory dish.

The Servings: 12
The Time to Prepare/Cook:
The Calories: 150
The Ingredients:
Red wine vinegar – 0.25 cup
Extra virgin olive oil – 0.75 cup
Parsley, fresh – 1 cup, packed
Oregano, fresh – 0.25 cup, packed
Garlic, chopped – 4 cloves
Sea salt – 1 teaspoon
Crushed red pepper flakes – 0.5 teaspoon
Cumin, ground – 0.5 teaspoon
Black pepper, ground – 0.25 teaspoon

The Instructions:
1. After washing your herbs, pull the leaves off of the stems, discarding the stems. The measurements for the herbs are for the leaves only, with the stems removed.
2. Add all of your ingredients into your food processor or blender and pulse the machine on high. You want to pulse the mixture until the contents are all chopped up and combined, but not completely smooth or pulverized.
3. Taste the chimichurri sauce and adjust the seasonings to your preference before using. You can make this sauce up to two days in advance.

Mango Habanero Sauce

This sweet and spicy sauce is the perfect addition to meat, seafood, fish, and tofu. It is just full of irresistible flavor! You can even add it to roasted vegetables, pizza, tacos, or use it as a dip for your favorite snacks.

The Servings: 6
The Time to Prepare/Cook: 10 minutes
The Calories: 27
The Ingredients:
Habanero peppers – 3
Mango – 1 cup
Water – 0.25 cup
Garlic – 3 cloves
Ginger, fresh, peeled – 0.5 inch root
Sea salt – 0.5 teaspoon
White vinegar – 0.5 cup
Lime juice – 2 tablespoons
Black pepper, ground – 0.25 teaspoon
The Instructions:
1. Add the water, habanero peppers, mango, garlic, and ginger into your blender and pulse until it is completely smooth. Transfer the mango and habanero mixture to a saucepan and warm it over low until hot. Stir in the seasonings and vinegar.
2. Continue heating the sauce until it begins to bubble and thicken, and then remove it from the heat. Stir in the lime juice. Use the mango habanero sauce immediately or allow it to cool before storing it in a jar in the fridge for later use.

Stir-Fry Sauce

This sauce is great for whenever you want to make stir-fry vegetables, but it is also great over meats, tofu, and rice. Enjoy this all-purpose stir-fry sauce whenever you feel the craving for East Asian take-out.

The Servings: 8
The Time to Prepare/Cook: 10 minutes
The Calories: 32
The Ingredients:
Date paste – 2 tablespoons
Sesame seed oil – 2 teaspoons
Garlic, minced – 3 cloves
Ginger, fresh, minced – 2 tablespoons
Cornstarch – 1 tablespoon
Red pepper flakes – 0.5 teaspoon
Low-sodium soy sauce – 0.33 cup
Vegetable broth – 0.5 cup
The Instructions:
1. Whisk together all of the stir-fry sauce ingredients until combined.
2. You can store the mixture in the fridge until ready to use, allowing it to heat and thicken with whatever ingredients you are cooking it with. Or, you can cook and thicken it in advance in a saucepan over medium heat until it boils and thickens.

Creamy Cauliflower Alfredo Sauce

You will be surprised by how delicious this Alfredo sauce is, despite being made with cauliflower! You can choose to make this sauce either with dairy milk, or dairy-free options such as soy milk. This makes it a great choice, as you can make it according to your specific needs.

The Servings: 10
The Time to Prepare/Cook: 15 minutes
The Calories: 58
The Ingredients:
Cauliflower florets – 6 cups
Garlic, minced – 8 cloves
Sea salt – 1 teaspoon
Vegetable broth – 7 cups
Extra virgin olive oil – 2 tablespoons
Black pepper, ground – 0.5 teaspoon
Milk of choice – 0.5 cup

The Instructions:
1. Add the garlic and extra virgin olive oil to a large skillet and allow it to sauté over medium until it is fragrant but not yet browned. Be careful to not burn the garlic. Remove the pan with the toasted garlic and oil from the heat and set it aside.
2. In a large pot, bring your vegetable broth to a boil. Once boiling, add in the cauliflower, cover the pot with a lid, and allow it to simmer over medium until the cauliflower is fork-tender—about seven to ten minutes.
3. Using a large kitchen utensil, transfer the tender cauliflower florets into your blender, along with one cup of the vegetable broth that they were simmered in. Add in your milk of choice, sautéed garlic and oil, and the seasonings.
4. Blend the cauliflower mixture on high speed until it is completely smooth and creamy. You can add more broth or milk if you want to adjust the thickness of the sauce. Be careful while blending, as the contents are hot. Taste the Alfredo sauce and adjust the seasonings to your taste before serving it over pasta or your choice of dishes.

Sweet and Spicy Marinade

This marinade is incredibly versatile! You will love it for vegetables, fish, seafood, or tofu. This makes the perfect amount of marinade for two servings, which means you can marinade about twelve ounces of meat in it.

The Servings: 2
The Time to Prepare/Cook: 5 minutes
The Calories: 199
The Ingredients:
Low-sodium soy sauce – 0.25 cup
Lemon juice – 2 tablespoons
Extra virgin olive oil – 2 tablespoons
Date paste – 2 tablespoons
Spicy brown mustard – 3 tablespoon
Garlic, minced – 4 cloves
Serrano pepper, diced – 1
Red pepper flakes – 0.5 teaspoon
Sea salt – 0.5 teaspoon
The Instructions:
1. Whisk together all of the sweet and spicy marinade ingredients until combined. Transfer the mixture to a container with a lid or a plastic bag; add in your meat, tofu, or vegetable of choice; and allow it to marinade in the fridge for at least thirty minutes before cooking.

Fresh Greek Marinade

This marinade is perfect for one pound of your choice of meat, seafood, fish, tofu, or vegetables. Whatever you choose to marinade in this, you are sure to love the fresh Greek flavor!

The Servings: 4
The Time to Prepare/Cook: 5 minutes
The Calories: 53
The Ingredients:
Lemon juice – 3 tablespoons
Extra virgin olive oil – 1.5 tablespoons
Red wine vinegar – 1 tablespoon
Garlic powder – 1 teaspoon
Sea salt – 0.5 teaspoon
Oregano, dried – 2 teaspoons
Paprika, ground – 0.25 teaspoon
Black pepper, ground – 0.25 teaspoon
The Instructions:
1. Whisk together all of the fresh Greek marinade ingredients in a kitchen mixing dish and then transfer the liquid to a container with a lid or a plastic bag. Add in one pound of your choice of meat or other ingredient options. Place the container in the fridge, allowing your ingredients to marinade for at least thirty minutes before cooking.

Brown Rice Gravy

This quick and easy brown gravy is gluten and dairy-free, making it perfect for nearly everyone on the anti-inflammatory diet! Since dairy and gluten are both common allergens, many people choose to or need to avoid them. But that doesn't mean you can't enjoy some of your favorite foods, such as delicious gravy.

When making this gravy, you can use whatever broth you want, whether beef, chicken, seafood, or vegetable. You can also use pan drippings, but keep in mind that pan drippings may be higher in sodium, so reduce the salt in the gravy if needed.

The Servings: 8
The Time to Prepare/Cook: 15 minutes
The Calories: 53
The Ingredients:
Brown rice flour – 2.5 tablespoons
Broth or pan drippings – 2 cups
Extra virgin olive oil – 2.5 tablespoons
Black pepper, ground – 0.25 teaspoon
Sea salt – 1

The Instructions:
1. Add your soil and brown rice flour into a large skillet to create a roux, and allow the brown rice flour roux to simmer over medium heat until it is lightly browned and toasted. Be careful to continue stirring the mixture so that it doesn't burn.
2. Once the roux smells toasted and nutty, slowly stir in the broth or pan drippings. Continue cooking while whisking constantly to avoid the formation of lumps. Allow the gravy to simmer and thicken until it reaches your desired thickness. Taste the gravy and add in the sea salt and pepper to taste before serving.

Dairy-Free Tzatziki Sauce

This fresh tzatziki sauce is a creamy Mediterranean staple, one which most people with dairy allergies are forced to live without. But, with this recipe, you can enjoy this delicious sauce on all of your favorite Mediterranean dishes, regardless of dairy allergies!

The Servings: 8
The Time to Prepare/Cook: 5 minutes
The Calories: 41
The Ingredients:
Tofu, soft – 1 pound
Apple cider vinegar – 1 teaspoon
Lemon juice – 3 tablespoons
Garlic, minced – 3 cloves
Black pepper, ground – 0.25 teaspoon
Water – 0.33 cup
English cucumber, grated – 1
Sea salt – 0.25 teaspoon
The Instructions:
1. Add all of the dairy-free tzatziki sauce ingredients, except for the English cucumber, to your blender or food processor and pulse until the tzatziki sauce is completely smooth. Transfer the mixture to a mixing dish.
2. Place the grated English cucumber inside a clean kitchen towel and fold up the corners to bundle the cucumber in the middle. Squeeze the bundle of cucumber to press out as much liquid as possible, discarding the liquid. Add the now-squeezed shredded cucumber to the mixing dish and stir it into the creamy tofu mixture. Enjoy the tzatziki sauce immediately, or store it in the fridge for up to a week.

Japanese Ginger Salad Dressing

This delicious and fresh dressing is inspired by the ginger salad dressings you might find at a Japanese restaurant. It's not only incredibly fresh and flavorful, it also has many powerful anti-inflammatory ingredients you will love!

The Servings: 10
The Time to Prepare/Cook: 10 minutes
The Calories: 116
The Ingredients:
Onion, diced – 0.25
Celery, diced- 2 stalks
Carrot, chopped – 1.5 cups
Ginger, peeled and grated – 2 tablespoons
Sea salt – 0.75 teaspoon
Rice wine vinegar – 3 tablespoons
Extra virgin olive oil – 0.5 cup
Low-sodium soy sauce – 0.25 cup
Date paste – 2 teaspoons
Black pepper, ground – 0.25 teaspoon
The Instructions:
1. Add all of your Japanese salad dressing ingredients to a food processor or blender and blend on high speed until the ginger dressing is creamy and smooth. Taste the Japanese salad dressing and adjust the seasoning to your preference. Serve the dressing over your salad of choice.

Strawberry Poppy Seed Vinaigrette

This vinaigrette makes an irresistible topping for any salad that is both sweet and savory. You can make it any time of the year that strawberries are available, but it is especially delicious when they are fresh in season.

The Servings: 4
The Time to Prepare/Cook: 5 minutes
The Calories: 88
The Ingredients:
Strawberries, chopped – 1 cup
Sea salt – 0.25 teaspoon
Red wine vinegar – 1 tablespoon
Extra virgin olive oil – 2 tablespoons
Date paste – 1 tablespoon
Poppy seeds – 2 teaspoons
The Instructions:
1. Add all of the strawberry vinaigrette ingredients, except the poppy seeds, into your blender and mix it on high until the strawberry vinaigrette is creamy and smooth. Add in the poppy seeds and quickly give the blender a couple small pulses just to combine without crushing all of the poppy seeds. Serve the vinaigrette over your salad of choice.

Green Goddess Salad Dressing

This dressing is perfect for whenever you want a dressing that is full of fresh flavor and herbs. If you want a great option for lunch, make yourself a large salad, topping it with this green goddess dressing and your favorite cut of lean meat.

The Servings: 6
The Time to Prepare/Cook: 5 minutes
The Calories: 34
The Ingredients:
Greek yogurt, plain, non-fat – 1 cup
Sea salt – 0.5 teaspoon
Mint, fresh – 0.25 cup
Parsley, fresh – 0.25 cup
Cilantro, fresh – 0.25 cup
Basil, fresh – 0.25 cup
Chives – 0.25 cup
Garlic, minced – 2 cloves
Black pepper, ground – 0.25 teaspoon
The Instructions:
1. Add all of the ingredients together into the food processor or blender and combine on high speed until completely smooth and creamy. Serve over your favorite fresh salads, grilled vegetables, or meats.

Thousand Island Dressing

For this dressing, how healthy it is depends on the ingredients you use. This means you want to use the best mayonnaise and ketchup you can find. If you are purchasing mayonnaise, try to find one made with a healthy oil, such as olive, avocado, safflower, or canola. You also want to use mayonnaise and ketchup without sugar. You can find a great recipe for anti-inflammatory ketchup in my other book, The Anti-Inflammatory Diet Action Plan.

The Servings: 12
The Time to Prepare/Cook: 5 minutes
The Calories: 176
The Ingredients:
Olive oil mayonnaise – 1 cup
Ketchup – 2 tablespoons
Onion, minced – 0.25 cup
Garlic minced – 1 clove
Lemon juice – 1 teaspoon
Sweet pickle relish – 2 tablespoons
Sea salt – 0.25 teaspoon
Paprika – 0.5 teaspoon

The Instructions:
1. In a kitchen mixing dish, whisk together all of the dressing recipes until well combined.
2. Transfer the thousand island dressing to a jar and store in the fridge for up to one week if using store-bought mayonnaise. If you are using homemade mayonnaise, you should use this dressing within one day.

Simple Mayonnaise

This mayonnaise is full of heart-healthy and anti-inflammatory oils without all the additives, meaning you can feel good about including it in your diet! Enjoy this mayonnaise alone to accompany your favorite burgers and sandwiches or use it to make other recipes such as dressings, dips, and sauces.

The Servings: 16
The Time to Prepare/Cook: 7 minutes
The Calories: 126
The Ingredients:
Egg, room temperature – 1
Lemon juice – 1 teaspoon
Sea salt – 0.25 teaspoon
White wine vinegar – 1 tablespoon
Dijon mustard – 1 tablespoon
Safflower or canola oil – 1 cup

The Instructions:
1. When preparing your mayonnaise, use a device for emulsifying that is appropriately sized for the amount of mayonnaise you are making. Otherwise, it could make it difficult to get your mayonnaise to emulsify. I recommend using a smaller food processing mixing dish attachment or an immersion blender.
2. Add your egg at room temperature to your small food processor's mixing dish or into a large cup that can accommodate your immersion blender
3. Pulse the egg with the device you are using for about twenty seconds. Add in the sea salt, white wine vinegar, and Dijon mustard before pulsing for another twenty seconds.
4. Use a spatula to scrape down the sides of your mixing dish or cup and then turn your food processor or immersion blender back on. While the motor is running, slowly drizzle in one-quarter of the oil. You want this to be an incredibly light drizzle so that it is only coming out in drops. Do not be hasty in this step, as trying to rush it can prevent the mayonnaise from properly emulsifying.
5. Continue running your food processor or immersion blender until the mayonnaise has emulsified (thickened) and then you can continue to add the remaining oil. Once the mayonnaise has emulsified, you can be a little more liberal at the speed of which you add the oil.
6. After all of the safflower oil has been poured in, scrape down the sides and bottom of the container with a spatula and then run the motor for about ten more seconds to finish combining all the ingredients evenly.
7. As this mayonnaise contains raw egg, you must use it within twenty-four hours of preparing it and be sure to keep the homemade mayonnaise well chilled.

Beverages

Green Ginger Smoothie

This green smoothie is great for when you want a breakfast or snack full of anti-oxidants and vital nutrients. While some green smoothies will use spinach, this one uses kale which is lower in oxalates. While the high oxalate content of spinach will often prevent the body from absorbing important nutrients, by using kale instead you can absorb more of the nutrients you are eating.

The Servings: 2
The Time to Prepare/Cook: 5 minutes
The Calories: 181
The Ingredients:
Mango, frozen – 1.5 cups
Kale, chopped – 2 cups
Dates, pitted – 2
Chia seeds – 2 tablespoons
Ginger, grated – 1 tablespoon
Lemon juice – 3 tablespoons
Water – 1.25 cup
The Instructions:
1. Add all of the green ginger smoothie ingredients into the blender, starting with the liquid followed by the kale, dates, chia seeds, ginger, and lastly the mango. Begin blending your smoothie until it is completely smooth, scrapping down the sides with a spatula if necessary.
2. You can serve this smoothie as two small servings or one large smoothie.

Chocolate Banana Smoothie

This smoothie is a great snack or breakfast when you don't have much time to sit down and eat or simply don't feel like eating in the mornings. Plus, the flavor is to die for!

The Servings: 3
The Time to Prepare/Cook: 5 minutes
The Calories: 368
The Ingredients:
Almond milk, unsweetened – 1 cup
Bananas, frozen – 2
Rolled oats – 0.5 cup
Greek yogurt, plain, non-fat – 0.5 cup
Almond extract – 0.125 teaspoon
Vanilla extract – 0.25 teaspoon
Date, pitted – 1
Cocoa powder – 2 tablespoons
Almond butter – 3 tablespoons
Chia seeds – 2 tablespoons
The Instructions:
1. Add all of the chocolate banana smoothie ingredients to the blender, starting with the almond milk and Greek yogurt, followed in order with the extracts, date, cocoa, almond butter, chia seeds, rolled oats, and bananas. Blend this mixture on high until it is completely smooth without any lumps. Scrape down the sides with a spatula as-needed. Serve while fresh and cold.

Tropical Detox Smoothie

This tropical smoothie is full of ingredients that are good for your health and your body's natural detox ability, allowing you to truly care for your body and its needs.

The Servings: 1
The Time to Prepare/Cook: 5 minutes
The Calories: 282
The Ingredients:
Pineapple, frozen – 0.5 cup
Peaches, frozen – 0.5 cup
Mango, frozen – 0.5 cup
Lemon juice – 3 tablespoons
Lemon zest – 1.5 teaspoons
Date, pitted – 1
Ginger, peeled and grated – 1 tablespoon
Chia seeds – 1 tablespoon
Almond milk – 0.75 cup
The Instructions:
1. Add all of your tropical detox smoothie ingredients to the blender and blend on high until it is completely smooth without and lumps, scraping down the sides with a spatula as-needed. Adjust the liquid amount to make it thinner, if desired, then serve while cold.

Peach Cobbler Smoothie

This smoothie is perfect for anyone who loves a good Southern classic peach cobbler, as the peaches, oats, and cinnamon will make you feel as if you are enjoying a frozen treat version of the dessert. But this smoothie is healthy enough to enjoy for any meal.

The Servings: 1
The Time to Prepare/Cook: 5 minutes
The Calories: 395
The Ingredients:
Rolled oats – 3 tablespoons
Cinnamon, ground – 1 teaspoon
Peach slices, frozen – 2 cups
Flaxseed, ground – 1 tablespoon
Almond milk, unsweetened – 1.25 cup
Vanilla extract – 0.25 teaspoon
Date, pitted – 1
The Instructions:
1.   Add all of the peach cobbler smoothie ingredients to your blender and allow it to blend on high speed until the contents are completely smooth without any lumps. You may need to scrape down the sides with a spatula from time to time. Enjoy this smoothie while freshly made and cold.

Matcha Antioxidant Smoothie

This smoothie has matcha in it, which is great for its powerful antioxidant properties, as well as providing you with a nice caffeine boost! Feel free to add more or less matcha, according to taste. When adding protein powder, use one that is as pure and natural as possible, such as one that is 100% egg white or soy protein isolate.

The Servings: 1
The Time to Prepare/Cook: 5 minutes
The Calories: 265
The Ingredients:
Banana – 0.5
Strawberries, hulled – 1 cup
Spinach – 1 cup
Matcha powder – 0.75 teaspoon
Protein powder – 1 serving
Almond milk, unsweetened – 1 cup
Ice – 0.75 cup

The Instructions:
1. Add all of the matcha antioxidant smoothie ingredients to your blender and allow it to blend on high speed until the antioxidant smoothie's contents are completely smooth without any lumps. You may need to scrape down the sides with a spatula from time to time. Enjoy this smoothie while freshly made and cold.

Chocolate Pudding Shake

This shake is inspired by recipes for vegan chocolate pudding, which contains avocado. It may seem wild to add avocado to a pudding shake, but believe me, you won't taste it! The avocado is a great addition, because while the flavor is completely covered up by chocolate, it provides the creaminess we all love and know from pudding. Not only that, but avocado has many great health benefits.

The Servings: 1
The Time to Prepare/Cook: 5 minutes
The Calories: 398
The Ingredients:
Almond milk, unsweetened – 1 cup
Banana – 1
Cocoa powder – 2 tablespoons
Avocado – 0.5
Date – 1
Vanilla extract – 1 teaspoon
Ice cube – 1 cup
The Instructions:
1.   Add all of the chocolate pudding shake ingredients to your blender and allow it to blend on high speed until the pudding shake's contents are completely smooth without any lumps. You may need to scrape down the sides with a spatula from time to time. Enjoy this smoothie while freshly made and cold.

Coffee Breakfast Smoothie

This shake is a great option to have for breakfast, as it has all the nutrients you need along with your morning cup of coffee! This means you can easily enjoy a healthy and energizing breakfast, no matter how busy you may be.

The Servings: 1
The Time to Prepare/Cook: 5 minutes
The Calories: 569
The Ingredients:
Black coffee, cool – 1 cup
Almond milk, unsweetened – 1 cup
Banana – 1
Rolled oats – 0.5 cup
Chia seeds – 1 tablespoon
Vanilla extract – 0.5 teaspoon
Dates, pitted – 2
Ice – 1 cup
The Instructions:
1. Add all of the coffee breakfast smoothie ingredients to your blender and allow it to blend on high speed until the coffee smoothie is completely smooth without any lumps. You may need to scrape down the sides with a spatula from time to time. Enjoy this smoothie while freshly made and cold.

Apple Pie Protein Smoothie

This apple pie protein smoothie is perfect for when you need a boost in protein, a delicious snack, or even want to enjoy it for dessert! The apple pie flavor is delicious and creamy, just like your favorite apple pie with ice cream.

The Servings: 2
The Time to Prepare/Cook: 5 minutes
The Calories: 257
The Ingredients:
Greek yogurt, plain, non-fat – 0.5 cup
Almond milk, unsweetened – 1 cup
Red apples, peeled and cored – 2
Banana, frozen – 1
Cinnamon, ground – 1 teaspoon
Nutmeg, ground – 0.125 teaspoon
Ginger, ground – 0.125 teaspoon
Cloves, ground – 0.125 teaspoon
Date, pitted – 1
Ice – 1 cup

The Instructions:
1. Add all of the ingredients for the apple pie protein smoothie to your blender and allow it to blend on high speed until the contents are completely smooth without any lumps. You may need to scrape down the sides with a spatula from time to time. Enjoy this smoothie while freshly made and cold.

Lemonade Sunshine Shake

This lemonade shake is creamy and tangy from the additions of yogurt and ginger, and the lemon flavor is extra potent as it not only has lemon juice, but lemon zest as well. This shake is the perfect treat to cool off with on a hot summer day.

The Servings: 1
The Time to Prepare/Cook: 5 minutes
The Calories: 240
The Ingredients:
Yogurt, plain, low-fat – 1 cup
Date paste – 2 tablespoons
Vanilla extract – 0.5 teaspoon
Lemon juice – 2 tablespoons
Lemon zest – 2 teaspoons
Ginger, peeled and grated – 1 tablespoon
Turmeric, ground – 0.125 teaspoon
Ice cubes – 1 cup
The Instructions:
1. Add all of the ingredients for the lemonade sunshine shake to your blender and allow it to blend on high speed until the lemonade shake is completely smooth without any lumps. You may need to scrape down the sides with a spatula from time to time. Enjoy this shake while freshly made and cold.

Summer Watermelon Cooler

This cooler is a great way to use up some watermelon to cool yourself off and stay hydrated on the hot days of summer. If you want an extra special treat for adults, you can even make it spiked with the addition of a little vodka—making it great for a summer night party.

The Servings: 2
The Time to Prepare/Cook: 5 minutes
The Calories: 99
The Ingredients:
Peach, sliced – 1
Watermelon, chopped – 3 cups
Ice
Mint for garnish
The Instructions:
1. Add all of the ingredients for the summer watermelon cooler to your blender and allow it to blend on high speed until the watermelon cooler is completely smooth without any lumps. You may need to scrape down the sides with a spatula from time to time. Enjoy this cooler while freshly made and cold.

ACV Detox Tea

While it may seem odd to make a drink with apple cider vinegar, you will find that it tastes really good! Just as adding a little vinegar to a sauce or meal can improve its flavor, the same is true of this drink. The ACV is perfectly balanced with other flavors and sweeteners, making it a sweet and tangy drink that is great for your health. Enjoy this regularly to promote better digestive and immune health. For best results, use raw apple cider vinegar, such as Bragg's.

The Servings: 1
The Time to Prepare/Cook: 5 minutes
The Calories: 22
The Ingredients:
Water, hot – 1 cup
Apple cider vinegar – 2 tablespoons
Date paste – 1 teaspoon
Cinnamon, ground – 0.25 teaspoon
Ginger, peeled and grated – 1 teaspoon
Lemon juice – 2 tablespoons
Cayenne pepper – 1 dash

The Instructions:
1. Heat your water in a kettle, saucepan, or microwave and then combine it with the remaining ingredients, stirring to dissolve the date paste and incorporate the seasonings. Allow the ACV detox tea to steep for a few minutes, so that it takes on the flavor of the spices.
2. Strain your through a fine mesh sieve and serve while warm. Alternatively, you could wait for the tea to cool and then serve it over ice for a nice cold drink.

Desserts

Gluten-Free Lemon Bars

These lemon bars are sweet and zesty, perfect for any dessert whether it is the end of the workday, your day off work, or for a special holiday party. You can even freeze these bars individually and thaw one out whenever you find yourself craving sweets.

The Servings: 12
The Time to Prepare/Cook: 40 minutes
The Calories: 144
The Crust Ingredients:
Almond flour – 1.5 cups
Coconut flour – 0.25 cup
Soybean oil – 0.33 cup
Lakanto monk fruit sweetener – 0.25 cup
Vanilla extract – 1 teaspoon
Sea salt – 0.25 teaspoon
The Filling Ingredients:
Coconut flour, sifted – 1 tablespoon
Lemon zest – 1 teaspoon
Lakanto monk fruit sweetener – 0.5 cup
Lemon juice – 0.75 cup
Eggs, whole – 3
Egg yolk – 1
The Instructions:
1. Warm your oven to a temperature of Fahrenheit 350 degrees and prepare a baking dish of eight-by-eight inches by lining it with kitchen parchment. You can alternatively grease the pan with your favorite light oil, but parchment is easier.
2. In a mixing dish, combine together all of your crust ingredients. This is best done with a fork, so that you can fully distribute the oil through the flours. Place the crust in the bottom of your lined baking dish and press it down to form an even layer. Place the baking dish in the oven, allowing it to partially bake for fifteen minutes while you prepare the lemon filling.
3. To combine the filling, whisk together the eggs until the egg whites are completely broken down into the yolks. Add in the lemon juice and zest along with the sweetener. Once combined, whisk in the sifted coconut flour until no lumps remain.
4. Once the crust has finished partially baking, remove it from the oven and pour the filling over the top. Reduce your oven's temperature to Fahrenheit 325 degrees and place the dish back into the middle of the oven. Allow it to bake until the filling is set, about twenty to twenty-two minutes. Keep in mind, the filling might still jiggle a bit.
5. Allow the gluten-free lemon bars to cool at room temperature before placing them in the fridge to chill for at least three hours. Slice and serve cold.

Cherry Crisp

This cherry crisp is sweet and nutty, making it irresistible. But you will especially love how effortless it is to make! Anyone can make this dessert, no matter how little experience they have in baking, if they only follow the recipe.

The Servings: 10
The Time to Prepare/Cook: 65 minutes
The Calories: 176
The Filling Ingredients:
Sweet cherries, pitted and halved – 1.5 pounds
Vanilla extract – 1 teaspoon
Lemon juice – 1 tablespoon
Lakanto monk fruit sweetener – 0.25 cup
Cornstarch – 2 tablespoons
The Topping Ingredients:
Almonds, raw – 0.66 cup
Almond flour – 1 cup
Shredded coconut, unsweetened – 0.5 cup
Cinnamon, ground – 1 teaspoon
Vanilla extract – 1 teaspoon
Sea salt – 0.25 teaspoon
Lakanto monk fruit sweetener – 0.25 cup
The Instructions:
1. Warm your oven to Fahrenheit 350 degrees and prepare a nine inch round baking pan or pie dish for your crisp.
2. Begin by making the topping of the crisp. To do this, you can make the topping by hand or with a food processor. To make it by hand, you want to chop the almonds up with a sharp knife until they are large crumb pieces. This is easiest done in a food processor. Once your almonds are chopped up, mix them together with the remaining topping ingredients until it forms a crumbly mixture. Place the crumble topping in the fridge to chill while you prepare your cherry filling.
3. In a mixing dish, toss together all of the filling ingredients until the cherries are evenly coated in the mixture. Spread the mixture of cherries into your prepared baking dish and then sprinkle the chilled crumble over the top of them. Sprinkle the crumble as evenly as possible, so that the entire top of is covered.
4. Place your crisp in the hot oven to bake until the cherries are bubbly and the crumble is golden-brown, about forty minutes. Remove the pan of cherry crisp from the oven and allow it to cool for just a few minutes before serving. If desired, you can add a dollop of sweetened yogurt over the top.

Peanut Butter Banana Oatmeal Cookies

These cookies are incredibly simple with only a few ingredients in them, making it easy to enjoy sweets even when the pantry is bare. Enjoy these cookies as a sweet treat on-the-go, allowing you to enjoy a healthy sweet treat even when those around you are eating inflammation-causing desserts.

The Servings: 8
The Time to Prepare/Cook: 20 minutes
The Calories: 283
The Ingredients:
Rolled oats – 2 cups
Natural peanut butter – 0.5 cup
Bananas, mashed – 2
Baking powder – 0.75 teaspoon
Sea salt – 0.5 teaspoon
Date paste – 1 tablespoon
Vanilla extract – 0.5 teaspoon

The Instructions:
1. Warm your oven to Fahrenheit 350 degrees and prepare two large baking sheets by coating them in kitchen parchment or silicone mats.
2. Use a fork to mash your bananas in a mixing dish before adding in the remaining cookie ingredients. Stir together until they are combined.
3. Using a spoon or a cookie scoop, divide the cookie dough into sixteen evenly-sized portions on the baking sheets, using your fingers to shape the dough into cookie shapes. Keep in mind, these will remain in the same shape when you take them out of the oven, so shape them exactly how you want them to turn out.
4. Place the baking pans in the middle of the oven and allow your cookies to bake until they are slightly browned and set, about fifteen minutes. Remove the pans from the oven and transfer the cookies to wire racks to cool.

Zucchini Brownies

These brownies contain grated zucchini. While you may not be able to taste the squash, it will provide a great texture to the brownies keeping them moist and tender. While these brownies don't call for nuts, you can easily add a cup of your favorite chopped nuts, if you like!

The Servings: 8
The Time to Prepare/Cook: 45 minutes
The Calories: 233
The Ingredients:
Oat flour – 1.5 cups
Cocoa – 0.5 cup
Lakanto monk fruit sweetener – 0.75 cup
Instant coffee – 1 teaspoon (optional)
Sea salt – 0.5 teaspoon
Baking soda – 0.25 teaspoon
Baking powder – 1 teaspoon
Vanilla extract – 1 teaspoon
Almond butter – 0.5 cup
Almond milk, unsweetened – 0.25 cup
Zucchini, shredded – 1.25 cups
Lily's stevia-sweetened chocolate chips – 0.5 cups

The Instructions:
1. Warm your oven to Fahrenheit 350 degrees and line a five-by-nine inch loaf pan with kitchen parchment or grease it with your favorite light oil.
2. In a mixing dish, stir together the oat flour, cocoa, monk fruit sweetener, instant coffee, sea salt, baking soda, and baking powder. Once combined, stir in the zucchini, almond milk, almond butter, and vanilla extract. Lastly, fold in the chocolate chips. If you are using nuts, add them in when you add the chocolate chips.
3. Place the loaf pan in the middle of your oven and allow it to bake for forty to forty-five minutes. You can bake the zucchini brownies a little less for extra fudgy brownies or a little more if you want more cake-like brownies.
4. Remove your dish of zucchini brownies from the oven and allow them to cool completely before slicing. While you may be tempted to eat them right away, this is an important step for them to set up since they are gluten-free. If you want the brownies to taste extra good, you can chill them in the fridge for a couple days, which will deepen the flavors.

www.ingramcontent.com/pod-product-compliance
Lightning Source LLC
Chambersburg PA
CBHW081117080526
44587CB00021B/3631